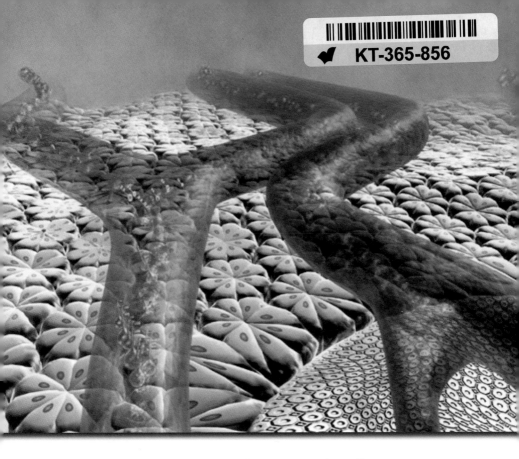

Hot Topics in Diabetes

Jiten Vora

Hot Topics in Diabetes

Editor: Jiten Vora

Publisher: Synergy
                       Synergy House
                       16 Petersham Road
                       Richmond
                       Surrey
                       TW10 6UW
                       www.synergymedical.co.uk

Cover image: Getty Images

ISBN: 978-1-897859-96-4

A catalogue record of this book is available from the British Library

This publication has been supported by an unrestricted educational grant from GSK.

Contributors

CJ Bailey, Professor and Head of Diabetes Research, Life and Health Sciences, Aston University, Birmingham, UK

J Betteridge, BSc, PhD, MD, FRCP, FAHA, Professor of Endocrinology and Metabolism, Royal Free and University College Medical School, London, UK

R Bilous, MD, FRCP, Professor of Clinical Medicine, Newcastle University Hon. Consultant Diabetes & Endocrinology, South Tees Acute Trust, Academic Centre, James Cook University Hospital, Middlesbrough, UK

CD Byrne, FRCP, FRCPath, PhD, Professor of Endocrinology and Metabolism, Southampton General Hospital, Southampton, UK

RM Cubbon, Leeds Institute of Genetics, Health and Therapeutics, University of Leeds, UK

PM Dodson, Associate Professor, Clinical Science Research Institute, Warwick Medical School, Consultant Physician, Medical Ophthalmology, Diabetes, Heart of England Foundation Trust, Bordesley Green East, Birmingham, UK

M Evans, MD, Consultant Diabetologist, Llandough Hospital, Cardiff, UK

AK Gupta, MBBS, MD, MSc, Clinical Research Fellow, International Centre for Circulatory Health, National Heart & Lung Institute, Imperial College London, UK

S Harding, FRCOphth MD, Consultant Ophthalmologist/Honorary Professor, St. Paul's Eye Unit, Royal Liverpool University Hospital, Liverpool, UK

L Holder, Department of Diabetes, Llandough Hospital, Cardiff, UK

MT Kearney, Professor of Cardiology, Leeds Institute of Genetics, Health and Therapeutics, The University of Leeds, UK

R Peter, Department of Diabetes, Llandough Hospital, Cardiff, UK

NR Poulter, Professor of Preventive Cardiovascular Medicine, International Centre for Circulatory Health, Imperial College London and St Mary's Hospital, London, UK

S Tesfaye, MD, FRCP, Consultant Physician and Honorary Professor of Diabetic Medicine (University of Sheffield), Royal Hallamshire Hospital, Sheffield, UK

S Thomas, MD, FRCP, Consultant in Diabetes and Endocrinology, Diabetes Centre, St Thomas' Hospital, Guy's & St Thomas' NHS Foundation Trust, London, UK

SH Wild, FRCP(Edin), FFPH, PhD, Senior Lecturer in epidemiology and public health, Public Health Sciences, University of Edinburgh, Teviot Place, Edinburgh, UK

Contents

Foreword

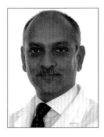

We live in exciting times in the world of diabetes, particularly in relation to the development of new therapies and systems for delivery of care. These are of course vital in relation to the expected worldwide explosion of diabetes, and at any given moment there is considerable information available to medical and paramedical staff who are involved in the care of people with diabetes. With a plethora of information and information sites, maintenance of a state-of-the-art knowledge becomes difficult.

This book, based on an idea created at the Annual Professional Conference of Diabetes UK, brings together experts in their fields who present brief chapters on diverse aspects of diabetes care that are currently considered 'hot'. I hope you will find the book a useful resource.

Publication of this book was made possible by an unrestricted educational grant from GlaxoSmithKline Pharmaceuticals and we are grateful for their support.

Dr Jiten Vora
Consultant Physician/Endocrinologist
Royal Liverpool University Hospitals
Liverpool
UK

The myocardium and acute myocardial infarction in diabetes

Dr Richard M Cubbon, Professor Mark T Kearney

Key points

- Diabetes significantly increases cardiovascular risk.
- The majority of acute myocardial infarction (AMI) sufferers exhibit abnormal glucose homeostasis if assessed comprehensively.
- Consensus guidelines support aggressive therapy, including tight glycaemic control, in patients with diabetes presenting with AMI.
- Despite improvements in medical therapy, patients with diabetes continue to experience high mortality rates.
- Novel treatments are needed to reduce cardiovascular risk in diabetes.

Introduction

It is now clear that we are in the midst of an epidemic of type 2 diabetes. The principal cause of death in patients with this complex disorder is cardiovascular disease (CVD). Most studies demonstrate that people with type 2 diabetes have up to three-fold increased risk of CVD. While the main cardiovascular complications of diabetes are micro- and macrovascular disease, it has also emerged that diabetes *per se* may have an impact on cardiovascular function leading to 'diabetic cardiomyopathy'. This review discusses:

1. Our current understanding of the pathophysiology and diagnosis of diabetic cardiomyopathy
2. Contemporary outcomes of patients with diabetes who have sustained an acute myocardial infarction (AMI).

Diabetic cardiomyopathy

The clustering of cardiovascular risk factors in patients with type 2 diabetes is well recognised. It is therefore not surprising that patients with type 2 diabetes are prone to the development of left ventricular (LV) dysfunction and chronic heart failure (CHF). Data from the Framingham Heart Study demonstrated that the prevalence of CHF in men and women with type 2 diabetes is increased at least two-fold.[1] While this is likely to be due, at least in part, to coronary artery disease (CAD) and hypertension, some patients with type 2 diabetes have LV dysfunction in the absence of these comorbidities. Hence the term diabetic cardiomyopathy first described by Rubler *et al.* over 30 years ago.[2] This is distinct from 'diabetic heart disease' which also encompasses cardiac disease related to the broad spectrum of cardiovascular insults associated with diabetes (Figure 1).

Figure 1: Diabetic heart disease

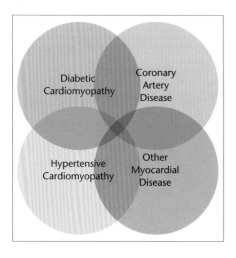

Diabetic cardiomyopathy is a clinical entity: supporting evidence

Cardiac biopsies from patients with type 2 diabetes have demonstrated a range of abnormalities in the absence of hypertension and CAD. Right ventricular biopsy specimens from patients with type 2 diabetes demonstrated myocyte hypertrophy and interstitial fibrosis.[3] Regan *et al.* demonstrated increased interstitial fibrosis and glycoprotein accumulation in autopsy specimens from normotensive diabetes patients without obstructive epicardial or intramural arterial disease.[4] Non-invasive techniques have supported these findings in larger cohorts. Ultrasonic integrated backscatter (a research based method of tissue ultrasound analysis) for example, correlates with tissue collagen content and is significantly elevated in patients with uncomplicated type 2 diabetes.[5]

Modern echocardiographic techniques can detect subtle abnormalities of LV function. This has highlighted the presence of myocardial dysfunction associated with type 2 diabetes, when hypertension and/or CAD are absent. Myocardial strain and strain-rate, markers of systolic function, are decreased in patients with isolated type 2 diabetes and are further diminished in the presence of hypertension.[5] Diastolic dysfunction, an abnormality of LV relaxation associated with an adverse prognosis,[6] is also detectable in type 2 diabetes patients. For example, Poirier *et al.* showed that 60% of patients with uncomplicated type 2 diabetes have abnormal mitral inflow Doppler waveforms (Figure 2), suggestive of mild (32%) to moderate (28%) diastolic dysfunction.[7] More sensitive tissue Doppler studies have suggested the prevalence of diastolic dysfunction in such patients to be as high as 75%.[8]

Pathophysiology

The functional and structural abnormalities observed in patients with uncomplicated type 2 diabetes provide compelling support for the concept of diabetic cardiomyopathy.

Figure 2: Mitral inflow patterns in LV diastolic dysfunction

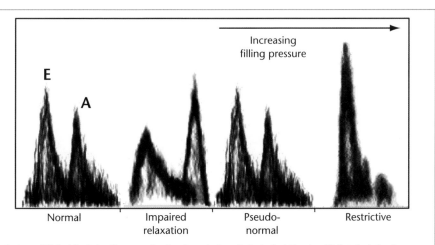

The features of LV diastolic dysfunction seen using Doppler evaluation of mitral valve inflow. In mild diastolic dysfunction, impaired LV relaxation reduces the velocity of early (E) flow and its deceleration; atrial (A) contribution to LV filling is increased. As diastolic dysfunction becomes moderate, increased left atrial pressures return the flow pattern to 'pseudo-normal'. With progressive deterioration in LV relaxation and compliance, filling pressures rise further resulting in predominant early flow which decelerates abruptly, denoted by a tall and steep E wave. Atrial contribution to LV filling is minimal in this 'restrictive' filling pattern.

Theories of mechanisms contributing to the development of diabetic cardiomyopathy include: hyperglycaemia, elevated free fatty acids, accelerated cardiac fibrosis, microvascular dysfunction and cardiac autonomic neuropathy; all are likely to contribute to some extent (Figure 3). For a more detailed discussion please refer to the excellent review of Fang et al.[9]

Figure 3: Pathophysiology of diabetic cardiomyopathy

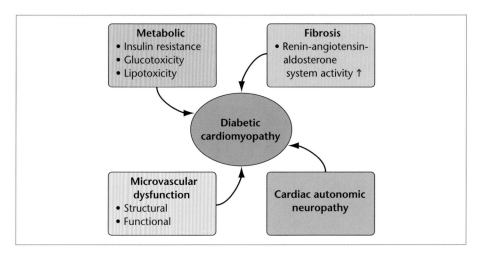

Suboptimal glycaemic control has been associated with systolic and diastolic dysfunction in patients with type 1 and type 2 diabetes. Furthermore, studies suggest administration of insulin can improve diastolic dysfunction and abnormal myocardial perfusion. In animal models of diabetes the myocardial capacity to utilise glucose also appears to be impaired, perhaps as a result of excess circulating free fatty acids leading to accumulation of toxic lipid metabolites. Such metabolic disturbances also appear to directly impair the efficiency of cardiac contraction. Moreover, generation of reactive oxygen species (ROS) and advanced glycosylation end-products (AGE) may result in endothelial dysfunction and enhanced interstitial fibrosis.

Correlating with pathological and radiological evidence of increased interstitial fibrosis, many pathophysiological processes associated with collagen deposition are also active in type 2 diabetes. In particular, the renin–angiotensin–aldosterone system (RAAS) appears to be up-regulated, and is well recognised to stimulate interstitial fibrosis. RAAS activity is also associated with increased apoptosis and necrosis of myocytes, fibroblasts and endothelial cells that may further stimulate myocardial fibrosis, so impairing systolic and diastolic function and possibly initiating a vicious cycle of cardiac functional decline.

The absence of epicardial CAD in some patients with diabetic cardiomyopathy, along with the frequent occurrences of renal, retinal and neural microvascular disease in type 2 diabetes, suggests myocardial microvascular disease may contribute to diabetic cardiomyopathy. Diabetic nephropathy certainly appears to be associated with the development of diabetic cardiomyopathy. Pathological studies also suggest structural abnormalities of myocardial microvessels are more common in type 2 diabetes. Consistent with this, studies have demonstrated impaired coronary flow reserve in selected patients with diabetes; this was associated with diastolic dysfunction.[10]

Investigation

Diabetic cardiomyopathy results in abnormalities of cardiac structure and function. Echocardiography, a cornerstone of cardiac investigation, is able to detect many of the subtle abnormalities of LV systolic and diastolic function. Simple Doppler assessment of mitral valve inflow can detect diastolic dysfunction in many patients with diabetes (Figure 2); tissue Doppler imaging (TDI) appears to add complimentary information and magnetic resonance imaging offers a further means of assessing the myocardial structure and function.[11]

Management of diabetic cardiomyopathy

Specific therapeutic interventions in diabetic cardiomyopathy are limited by a lack of definition and awareness of the disorder itself, resulting in few patients being identified as sufferers early in the disease. Furthermore, separating this condition from co-existing hypertensive and ischaemic heart disease is challenging.

The complex pathogenesis of the syndrome suggests a simple solution is unlikely. However, many of the key pathophysiological processes highlighted are addressed to some extent by evidence-based therapies targeted at other diabetic complications. These strategies should be used in all patients whilst research continues. It may be that screening of high-risk groups, such as those with diabetic nephropathy, offers the simplest way of identifying people who may benefit from treatment in future clinical trials.

Glycaemic control has been shown to improve markers of diastolic dysfunction associated with diabetes.[12] Provision of RAAS antagonists is also accepted to reduce cardiovascular and renal events in type 2 diabetes; given the pro-fibrotic effects of these substances, RAAS antagonism is also likely to be beneficial in diabetic cardiomyopathy.[13]

The compound effects of diabetic and ischaemic heart disease suggest that targeting the latter, for which the evidence base is greater, could improve outcomes; equally, blood pressure control is important. More investigational techniques such as collagen cross-link breakers (agents that retard glycation-dependent collagen cross-linking) show early promise, although they are not ready for wide-scale adoption.[14] Inflammation and oxidant stress are also likely to play a role in future therapeutic strategies, aiming to improve cardiac microvascular function, neuropathy and fibrosis.

Diabetic cardiomyopathy: key points

- Diabetic cardiomyopathy is a real and common entity.
- Abnormalities of LV systolic and diastolic function are caused by multiple pathophysiological processes.
- Echocardiography, using modern techniques, provides the most practical means of diagnosis and assessment.
- The evidence base for management is limited, but should focus on improving glycaemic control, insulin sensitivity and hypertension (especially with RAAS antagonists).
- LV systolic dysfunction should be managed according to globally accepted guidelines.
- LV diastolic dysfunction requires heart rate control to augment LV filling time along with judicious use of diuretics.

AMI in patients with diabetes

The citation classic from Stephen Haffner published in 1998 suggested that patients with type 2 diabetes have the same risk of a cardiovascular event as an individual without diabetes who has sustained an AMI.[15] While some but not all studies support this finding, at least in part as a result of Stephen Haffner's report, type 2 diabetes is now classed as a CVD equivalent. More recently Gillian Booth and colleagues published a large retrospective cohort study using provincial health claims to identify all adults with (n ≈ 380,000) and without (n >9,000,000) diabetes in Ontario Canada.[16] These investigators demonstrated that the transition to high-risk for cardiovascular events, defined as an event-rate equivalent to a 10-year risk of 20% or more, occurred at a substantially younger age in people with diabetes than those without. As a result Booth *et al.* suggested that diabetes confers an equivalent cardiovascular risk to that of aging 15 years.

Over the last two decades major advances have been made in our understanding of the pathophysiology of CAD and AMI. As a result, therapies for patients sustaining an AMI have also developed significantly. Randomised, controlled trials have established pharmacological intervention or percutaneous reperfusion as important treatments in the acute phase of an AMI and, more recently, it has been suggested that metabolic control may also be important in patients with hyperglycaemia admitted with an AMI.[17] Moreover, an array of secondary preventative pharmacological agents such as angiotensin-converting enzyme (ACE) inhibitors, β-adrenoceptor antagonists (β-blockers), HMGCoA-reductase inhibitors (statins) and aspirin have become integral to treatment algorithms for patients after an AMI.

It is becoming increasingly evident that a substantial proportion of patients admitted with an AMI have type 2 diabetes or impaired glucose tolerance (IGT). Norhammar *et al.* demonstrated in a series of patients admitted with AMI that in patients with a random glucose less than 11.1 mmol/l, one third have overt diabetes and a further one third IGT at 3 months post-discharge.[18] Consensus guidelines from the European Society of Cardiology summarise much of the pertinent research regarding the management of AMI (and other cardiovascular disease) in the setting of diabetes.[19] Essentially, these support aggressive medical therapy (as per high-risk patients without diabetes) with early risk stratification and prompt use of revascularisation where appropriate. The issue of intravenous insulin use peri-AMI requires further clarification after the contrasting results of the DIGAMI studies,[20,21] though methodological differences between the studies may well explain these issues. Current expert opinion continues to favour strict glycaemic control using insulin infusions in patients with AMI and diabetes.[19]

The effect of contemporary therapies on the outcome of patients with diabetes suffering an AMI is unclear. In view of the large proportion of patients admitted to hospital with an AMI, who suffer from diabetes or are glucose intolerant, clarity on this matter is required. We recently examined the temporal changes in short- and long-term mortality in patients with and without diabetes who have suffered an AMI. To do this we used two very well characterised groups of patients recruited in the Evaluation of Methods and Management of Acute Coronary Events (EMMACE)-1 and EMMACE-2 studies.[22] These prospective cohort studies examined outcomes in consecutively admitted, unselected patients with confirmed acute coronary syndromes in multiple adjacent hospitals. Patients were recruited over a 3-month period in 1995 in EMMACE-1 and a 6-month period in EMMACE-2. Baseline characteristics, inpatient and discharge treatment were recorded.

This analysis gave us the opportunity to assess: changes in mortality in patients suffering from AMI in a well-defined geographical area; use of secondary prevention therapies; and changes in characteristics of patients with and without diabetes admitted with an AMI. In order to allow direct comparison of cohorts we selected validated cases of AMI based on the World Health Organisation criteria (two of: ischaemic chest pain; cardiac enzyme or biomarker elevation; serial electrocardiographic changes).

Over the period between 1995 and 2003 the prevalence of diabetes in patients with AMI increased from 12.5% to 16.6% (p<0.001). The mean age of patients with diabetes remained unchanged but was slightly greater than the patients without diabetes. As expected the provision of secondary prevention therapies increased substantially (Table 1). ACE inhibitor, β-blocker, statin and aspirin use was similar in patients with diabetes and those without. Mortality data were of particular interest in view of the pleasing uptake of evidence-based secondary prevention therapies. When comparing early mortality there was an impressive improvement, particularly in patients with diabetes (40% relative reduction in 30-day mortality between 1995 and 2003; p = 0.006). However, despite evidence-based therapies these improvements were not sustained at 18 months in patients with diabetes. As a result there was no significant improvement in mortality for patients with diabetes, whereas overall mortality at 18 months improved in patients without diabetes (14.6% relative improvement).

Table 1: Patient characteristics in the EMMACE-1 and -2 studies[22]

	Diabetes		No diabetes	
	EMMACE-1	EMMACE-2	EMMACE-1	EMMACE-2
Age (years)	71.0	71.4	69.7	69.6
Male (%)	53.4	60.3	64.6	64.4
Hypertension (%)	37.1	57.1*	28.4	39.9*
Heart failure (%)	11.8	8.6	7.8	5.2
IHD (%)	55.2	62.0	46.5	41.8
Antiplatelet agent (%)	65.6	86.3*	73.4	85.8*
Statin (%)	7.2	78.7*	7.0	80.6*
ACE inhibitor (%)	40.3	73.5*	30.7	64.7*
Beta-blocker (%)	28.1	62.3*	37.3	66.1*

Patient characteristics and use of secondary prevention therapies in patients with and without diabetes sustaining an AMI in 1995 and 2003.
* denotes p<0.05 between diabetes status groups. IHD - Ischaemic heart disease.

A number of factors could have contributed to the disappointing results seen in patients with diabetes. Outcome after an AMI is probably related to the extent of myocardial damage sustained during the index event and, in the longer term, due to recurrent vascular events. Of interest in our 2003 cohort there was no difference in Killip class (a measure of acute heart failure severity) or cardiac enzymes (in fact the patients with diabetes had a smaller rise in creatine kinase). This raises the intriguing possibility that patients with diabetes admitted with an AMI have a lower cardiac reserve than patients without diabetes; the role of diabetic cardiomyopathy in outcomes after an AMI, which we discussed earlier in this article, warrants attention.

Mortality in the longer term is predominantly thought to be due to recurrent ischaemic events. It is now becoming well accepted that patients with diabetes have different atherosclerotic plaque composition,[23] and a markedly pro-atherosclerotic environment compared with patients without diabetes. In our comparison of the EMMACE studies there was a greater increase in the proportion of AMI patients without ST-segment elevation in the population with diabetes. Non-ST-segment elevation AMI has been associated with a poorer long-term prognosis than AMI with ST-segment elevation.[24] It may be that targeting more novel risk factors such as oxidative stress and systemic/vascular inflammation is necessary to improve outcomes after an AMI in patients with diabetes.[25]

Conclusion

Diabetes and cardiovascular disease are inextricably linked through common pathophysiological pathways. Given the burgeoning prevalence of obesity and caloric excess we can expect to witness an epidemic of type 2 diabetes, often with cardiovascular co-morbidity. Our understanding of this inter-relationship continues to evolve, as highlighted by our developing understanding of diabetic cardiomyopathy as an entity. Furthermore, we are beginning to understand the importance of novel pathophysiological pathways in enhancing atherosclerotic progression in diabetes. Management strategies targeting these factors are likely to be crucial if we are to improve the persistent, dismal cardiovascular outcome of patients with diabetes.

References

1. Kannell WB, Hjortland M, Castelli WP. Role of diabetes in congestive heart failure: The Framingham study. *Am J Cardiol* 1974; **34**: 29–34.

2. Rubler S, Dlugash J, Yuceoglu YZ *et al.* New type of cardiomyopathy associated with diabetic glomerulosclerosis. *Am J Cardiol* 1972; **30**: 595–602.

3. Shin-ichi N, Akira G, Norihiko S *et al.* Quantitative approach to the histopathology of the biopsied right ventricular myocardium in patients with diabetes mellitus. *Heart Vessels* 1985; **1**: 43–7.

4. Regan TJ, Lyons MM, Ahmed SS *et al.* Evidence for cardiomyopathy in familial diabetes mellitus. *J Clin Invest* 1977; **60**: 885–99.

5. Fang ZY, Yuda S, Anderson V *et al.* Echocardiographic detection of early diabetic myocardial disease. *J Am Coll Cardiol* 2003; **41**: 611–17.

6. MacCarthy PA, Kearney MT, Nolan J *et al.* Prognosis in heart failure with preserved left ventricular systolic function: prospective cohort study. *BMJ* 2003; **327**: 78–9.

7. Poirier P, Bogaty P, Garneau C *et al.* Diastolic dysfunction in normotensive men with well-controlled type 2 diabetes: Importance of maneuvers in echocardiographic screening for preclinical diabetic cardiomyopathy. *Diabetes Care* 2001; **24**: 5–10.

8. Boyer JK, Thanigaraj S, Schechtman KB, Perez JE. Prevalence of ventricular diastolic dysfunction in asymptomatic, normotensive patients with diabetes mellitus. *Am J Cardiol* 2004; **93**: 870–5.

9. Fang ZY, Prins JB, Marwick TH. Diabetic cardiomyopathy: Evidence, mechanisms, and therapeutic implications. *Endocr Rev* 2004; **25**: 543–67.

10. Strauer BE, Motz W, Vogt M, Schwartzkopff B. Impaired coronary flow reserve in NIDDM: A possible role for diabetic cardiopathy in humans. *Diabetes* 1997; **46**: S119–24.

11. Thomas HM. Identification of diabetic cardiomyopathy with cardiac magnetic resonance imaging. *Int J Card Imaging* 2006; **22**: 91–2.

12. von Bibra H, Hansen A, Dounis V *et al.* Augmented metabolic control improves myocardial diastolic function and perfusion in patients with non-insulin dependent diabetes. *Heart* 2004; **90**: 1483–4.

13. Lim HS, MacFadyen RJ, Lip GYH. Diabetes mellitus, the renin-angiotensin-aldosterone system, and the heart. *Arch Intern Med* 2004; **164**: 1737–48.

14. Liu J, Masurekar MR, Vatner DE *et al.* Glycation end-product cross-link breaker reduces collagen and improves cardiac function in aging diabetic heart. *Am J Physiol Heart Circ Physiol* 2003; **285**: H2587–91.

15. Haffner SM, Lehto S, Ronnemaa T *et al.* Mortality from coronary heart disease in subjects with type 2 diabetes and in nondiabetic subjects with and without prior myocardial infarction. *N Engl J Med* 1998; **339**: 229–34.

16. Booth GL, Kapral MK, Fung K, Tu JV. Relation between age and cardiovascular disease in men and women with diabetes compared with non-diabetic people: a population-based retrospective cohort study. *Lancet* 2006; **368**: 29–36.

17. Malmberg K, Ryden L, Efendic S *et al.* Randomized trial of insulin-glucose infusion followed by subcutaneous insulin treatment in diabetic patients with acute myocardial infarction (DIGAMI study): effects on mortality at 1 year. *J Am Coll Cardiol* 1995; **26**: 57–65.

18. Norhammar A, Tenerz A, Nilsson G *et al.* Glucose metabolism in patients with acute myocardial infarction and no previous diagnosis of diabetes mellitus: a prospective study. *Lancet* 2002; **359**: 2140–4.

19. Task FM, Ryden L, Standl E *et al.* Guidelines on diabetes, pre-diabetes, and cardiovascular diseases: executive summary: The Task Force on Diabetes and Cardiovascular Diseases of the European Society of Cardiology (ESC) and of the European Association for the Study of Diabetes (EASD). *Eur Heart J* 2007; **28**: 88–136.

20. Malmberg K, Ryden L, Wedel H *et al.* Intense metabolic control by means of insulin in patients with diabetes mellitus and acute myocardial infarction (DIGAMI 2): effects on mortality and morbidity. *Eur Heart J* 2005; **26**: 650–61.

21. Malmberg K, Ryden L, Efendic S *et al.* Randomized trial of insulin-glucose infusion followed by subcutaneous insulin treatment in diabetic patients with acute myocardial infarction (DIGAMI Study): Effects on mortality at 1 year. *J Am Coll Cardiol* 1995; **26**: 57–65.

22. Cubbon RM, Wheatcroft SB, Grant PJ *et al.* Temporal trends in mortality of patients with diabetes mellitus suffering acute myocardial infarction: a comparison of over 3000 patients between 1995 and 2003. *Eur Heart J* 2007; **28**: 540–5.

23. Burke AP, Kolodgie FD, Zieske A *et al.* Morphologic findings of coronary atherosclerotic plaques in diabetics: A postmortem study. *Arterioscler Thromb Vasc Biol* 2004; **24**: 1266–71.

24. Allen LAM, O'Donnell CJM, Camargo CAJ *et al.* Comparison of long-term mortality across the spectrum of acute coronary syndromes. *Am Heart J* 2006; **151**: 1072–8.

25. Enzo B. The metabolic syndrome and cardiovascular disease. *Ann Med* 2006; **38**: 64–80.

Lipids and diabetes

Professor John Betteridge

Key points

- Diabetic dyslipidaemia is an important risk factor for cardiovascular disease (CVD) in diabetes and is open to effective therapeutic intervention.
- The major therapeutic target is low-density lipoprotein (LDL)-cholesterol.
- Robust randomised, controlled trials have demonstrated unequivocal benefit with statin drugs in the primary and secondary prevention of CVD.
- More intensive LDL-cholesterol lowering is associated with further CVD benefit.
- Recent guidelines have revised the target LDL-cholesterol down to 2 mmol/l on the basis of recent trial data, and this new target should be incorporated into the overall management of patients with diabetes.

Introduction

Cardiovascular disease (CVD) remains the most important cause of morbidity and mortality in patients with diabetes.[1] This high-risk population is more likely to suffer a fatal event as the first manifestation of myocardial infarction (MI) or stroke, making primary prevention a priority. The pathogenesis of atherosclerosis-related disease is multi-factorial and dyslipidaemia, an important risk factor, is common and open to therapeutic intervention.[2]

Pharmacological intervention is supported by robust, large, randomised, controlled clinical trials (RCTs) of primary and secondary CVD prevention. RCTs with statin drugs have demonstrated unequivocal benefit in reducing major coronary events, stroke and overall mortality.

Recently, the Joint British Societies (JBS) updated their guidance on CVD prevention (JBS2).[3] After reviewing evidence from more recent RCTs that showed that more clinical benefit was achieved with more intensive cholesterol lowering, the guideline committee recommended that the goals of therapy for total cholesterol and low-density lipoprotein (LDL)-cholesterol targets should be revised and lowered from 5 and 3 mmol/l, suggested in the previous joint guidelines,[4] to 4 and 2 mmol/l, respectively. However, these new targets have been criticised in some quarters, most likely due to the increased cost of implementation, as the use of more potent statins or combination therapy would be required more frequently and these drugs are not yet off-patent.

In this chapter, evidence from RCTs for the new treatment targets will be discussed in relation to patients with diabetes who are at high risk of CVD. In this author's opinion, a strong case can be made for the adoption of the more intensive targets. Knowledge gained from clinical science should stand clear and true and not be obscured by those who seek to restrict health-care costs. If well-researched and beneficial clinical treatment cannot be afforded by the health-care system, then that fact should be stated clearly in an honest and open manner. Sadly, this does not seem to be the case and the various attacks on the integrity and balance of the guideline writers who laboured to produce the JBS2 is inappropriate and strikes at the very foundation of clinical science.

LDL cholesterol and vascular risk in diabetes

Diabetic dyslipidaemia is characterised by moderately raised triglycerides, low high-density lipoprotein (HDL) cholesterol, and the accumulation of cholesterol-enriched remnant lipoprotein particles.[5] Total and LDL-cholesterol concentrations are not particularly raised in patients with diabetes and mainly reflect those of the background population; however, these parameters remain important risk factors. In men screened for the Multiple Risk Factor Intervention Trial (MRFIT), total cholesterol was an important determinant of CVD mortality in patients with diabetes, as in those without, and for a given cholesterol concentration, CVD risk was two- to three-fold higher.[6] LDL cholesterol was the best predictor of MI in the United Kingdom Prospective Diabetes Study (UKPDS); based on the observational epidemiology, a 1 mmol/l increase in LDL is associated with a 57% increased risk.[7]

There are important qualitative changes in LDL particle distribution in diabetic dyslipidaemia which are likely to increase its atherogenicity.[5] The density distribution is shifted to smaller, denser particles – so-called small, dense LDL. These particles have less polar lipid, leading to altered surface accessibility of apolipoprotein (apo) B, the major apoprotein of LDL. These segments show increased binding affinity to glycosaminoglycans, suggesting these particles are more likely to stick in the arterial wall. Small, dense LDL is also more susceptible to oxidation and it is oxidised LDL which is central to many of the processes of atherogenesis.[8,9] LDL cholesterol underestimates the number of LDL particles when they are small and dense. There is one molecule of apo B per LDL particle and measurement of plasma apo B helps to identify the presence of small, dense LDL, as the level will be higher than expected for the LDL-cholesterol concentration.[10] In the future, it is likely that the apo B measurement will be used more in clinical practice.

LDL cholesterol lowering with statins

Statins are specific, competitive inhibitors of HMG-coenzyme A reductase, the enzyme that catalyses the major, rate-determining step in cholesterol synthesis. In cell systems these compounds inhibited cholesterol synthesis at nanomolar concentrations,[11] resulting in increased LDL-receptor expression and therefore increased uptake of LDL. The statins have proved to be highly effective in lowering plasma LDL, in addition to being safe and well tolerated.[11]

Secondary prevention trials

In The Scandinavian Simvastatin Survival Study (4S),[12] patients with established coronary heart disease (CHD) and raised plasma cholesterol concentrations (5.5–8 mmol/l) were randomly allocated to placebo or treatment with simvastatin 20–40 mg/day to reduce plasma LDL cholesterol to <5 mmol/l or placebo. Patients receiving simvastatin maintained a 35% reduction in LDL cholesterol during the course of the study, and demonstrated a 30% reduction in overall mortality (hazard ration (HR) 0.7; 95% confidence interval (CI): 0.58–0.85; p<0.0003). In addition, significant reductions were seen in all coronary events.[12] A *post hoc* analysis in the subgroup of patients with diabetes, showed that the lipid changes were similar to those observed overall. This analysis demonstrated that patients with diabetes and CHD are at very high risk, as approximately half the patients in the placebo group suffered a major event during the study period. In the simvastatin group, there was a 55% reduction in CVD events (p = 0.002). The numbers were too small to assess the effect on overall mortality, although there was a 47%, non-significant reduction.[13]

In a further analysis, additional patients with diabetes (total n = 483) were identified on the basis of a baseline fasting glucose ≥7.0 mmol/l.[14] In addition, 678 patients were identified with impaired fasting glucose (IFG), defined as glucose levels between 6.1 and 6.9 mmol/l. There was a significant reduction in major CHD events of 42% with simvastatin in the enlarged diabetes cohort (HR 0.58; 95% CI: 0.42–0.81; p<0.001). The 28% reduction in overall mortality did not reach statistical significance. In the group with IFG, the 43% reduction in overall mortality was significant (HR 0.57; 95% CI: 0.31–0.91; p<0.02).[14]

Subsequent studies of secondary CVD prevention, such as Cholesterol And Recurrent Events (CARE),[15] Long-term Intervention with Pravastatin in Ischaemic Disease (LIPID)[16] and Heart Protection Study (HPS)[17,18] confirmed the findings of 4S in CHD patients with a wide range of cholesterol concentrations. In these studies, the reduction in CVD events proved to be similar in subgroups of patients with diabetes.

Intensive statin therapy

In the Cholesterol Treatment Trialists' (CTT) Collaboration meta-analysis of 14 RCTs involving 90,056 participants taking statins, the proportional reduction in CVD events was directly related to the degree of LDL cholesterol lowering.[19] This analysis suggested that if LDL cholesterol lowering could be targeted more intensively, more clinical benefit could be achieved. This hypothesis is particularly important to test in a population with diabetes, given the high residual risk observed despite conventional statin therapy. For instance, in HPS, residual risk in patients with diabetes and CVD, on statin therapy was higher than those with CVD but no diabetes on placebo.[18]

In the Pravastatin or Atorvastatin Evaluation and Infection Therapy (PROVE-IT) trial, standard statin therapy (pravastatin 40 mg/day) was compared with intensive therapy (atorvastatin 80 mg/day) in patients within 10 days of acute coronary syndrome.[20] The more intensive LDL cholesterol lowering with atorvastatin (mean LDL 1.6 mmol/l achieved) was associated with a highly significant (p = 0.005) 16% risk reduction in cardiovascular events compared with pravastatin (mean LDL 2.46 mmol/l). In a pre-specified analysis of the patients with diabetes included in the PROVE-IT trial,[21] the rate of acute cardiac events (death, MI, and unstable angina requiring hospitalisation) was much higher in patients with diabetes but was reduced by intensive vs. standard therapy similarly in patients with (21.1% vs. 26.6%; HR 0.75; p = 0.03) and without diabetes (14% vs. 18%; HR 0.76; p = 0.002), (p-interaction = 0.97). In patients with diabetes, 55 events were saved per 1,000 patients treated compared with 44 in those without diabetes.[21]

The Treat to New Targets (TNT) Trial has reported on the effects of intensive statin therapy (atorvastatin 80 mg/day) compared with standard therapy (atorvastatin 10 mg/day) in patients with stable CHD.[22] CHD patients with LDL cholesterol 3.4–6.5 mmol/l, and plasma triglycerides ≤6.8 mmol/l, entered an 8-week run-in treatment phase with open-label atorvastatin 10 mg/day. If an LDL-cholesterol concentration of <3.4 mmol/l was achieved, patients were randomised to either atorvastatin 10 mg/day or 80 mg/day. The primary end-point was a composite of CHD death, non-fatal, non-procedure-related MI, resuscitation after cardiac arrest and fatal or non-fatal stroke. Intensive therapy (mean LDL cholesterol 2.0 mmol/l) was associated with a 22% risk reduction (HR 0.78; 95% CI: 0.69–0.89; p<0.001) compared with standard therapy (mean LDL cholesterol 2.6 mmol/l). In the diabetes subgroup in TNT, mean LDL cholesterol was 2.5 mmol/l in the intensive-therapy group compared with 2.0 mmol/l in the standard-therapy group, and this was associated with a 25% risk reduction in major cardiovascular events (HR 0.75; 95% CI: 0.58–0.97; p = 0.026).[23]

On the basis of the new information discussed above, the guidelines of the US Adult Treatment Panel III were updated to include an optional, more intensive goal of therapy in those at highest risk, namely LDL cholesterol <1.8 mmol/l.[24] This target has also been advocated in the recent report of the Joint Task Force on Diabetes and Cardiovascular Disease of the European Society of Cardiology and European Association for the Study of Diabetes.[25]

A recent meta-analysis of trials of more intensive statin therapy compared with conventional therapy included 27,548 subjects in four major studies, two in stable coronary disease (TNT and Incremental Decrease in End Points Through Aggressive Lipid-Lowering (IDEAL)) and two in acute coronary syndrome (PROVE-IT and Aggrastat® to Zocor® trial (A-to-Z)).[26] This analysis strongly supports the concept that there is additional clinical benefit from more intensive therapy, as demonstrated by a

16% odds ratio reduction in coronary death or MI (HR 0.84; 95% CI: 0.77–0.91; p = 0.00003). No difference was observed in total or non-cardiovascular mortality (Table 1).

Table 1: Meta-analysis of cardiovascular outcomes – intensive vs moderate statin therapy.[26]

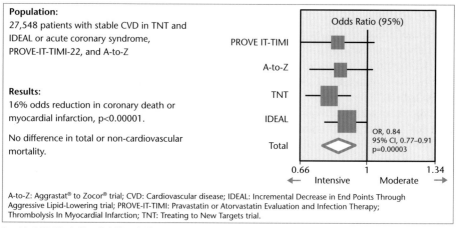

Population: 27,548 patients with stable CVD in TNT and IDEAL or acute coronary syndrome, PROVE-IT-TIMI-22, and A-to-Z	Odds Ratio (95%)
Results: 16% odds reduction in coronary death or myocardial infarction, p<0.00001. No difference in total or non-cardiovascular mortality.	OR, 0.84 95% CI, 0.77–0.91 p=0.00003

A-to-Z: Aggrastat® to Zocor® trial; CVD: Cardiovascular disease; IDEAL: Incremental Decrease in End Points Through Aggressive Lipid-Lowering trial; PROVE-IT-TIMI: Pravastatin or Atorvastatin Evaluation and Infection Therapy; Thrombolysis In Myocardial Infarction; TNT: Treating to New Targets trial.

Copyright © 2006 Elsevier Biomedical. Adapted with permission from Cannon *et al.* *J Am Coll Cardiol* 2006; **48**: 438–45.

Primary prevention trials

Given the high risk of CVD in patients with diabetes, together with a higher mortality associated with the first event, primary prevention with lipid lowering is an important component of global-preventive strategies in patients with diabetes.

Large cohorts of patients with diabetes without established CVD were included in HPS[18] and the Anglo–Scandinavian Cardiac Outcomes Trial – Lipid-Lowering Arm (ASCOT–LLA).[27] In ASCOT–LLA, 10 mg of atorvastatin was compared with placebo in 10,305 patients with hypertension and non-fasting total cholesterol of ≤6.5 mmol/l, of whom 2,532 had type 2 diabetes. Atorvastatin therapy was associated with a 36% reduction in the primary endpoint of non-fatal MI and fatal CHD after a median follow up of 3.3 years (the trial was stopped early because the pre-specified stopping criteria were achieved). Tests for heterogeneity showed that those with diabetes (n = 2,532) responded in a similar way although there were too few events (n = 84) to assess reliably the effect in the subgroup alone. In HPS there were 2,912 patients with diabetes without symptomatic vascular disease.[18] First major vascular events occurred in 135 (9.3%) patients receiving simvastatin 40 mg/day versus 196 (13.5%) placebo patients – a risk reduction of 33% (p = 0.0003) with simvastatin. It was estimated that a major vascular event could be prevented in approximately 45 patients per 1,000 treated.

The Collaborative Atrovastatin Diabetes Study (CARDS) was the first trial to specifically study a type 2 diabetes population. In this RCT, atorvastatin 10 mg/day was compared with placebo in a population of patients with type 2 diabetes (aged 40–75 years) and LDL cholesterol ≤4.14 mmol/l, plasma triglycerides ≤6.78 mmol/l, and one other CVD risk factor: hypertension, retinopathy, proteinuria or cigarette smoking.[28] The trial was event-driven and was expected to terminate in 2005 when 304 events had accumulated. However, after the second pre-planned interim analysis the data and safety-monitoring committee advised that the stopping criteria had been fulfilled and the trial was terminated early with 210 events. The primary event was time to first major CVD event (a composite of acute coronary events, coronary revascularisation and fatal or non-fatal stroke). The absolute reduction in LDL cholesterol with atorvastatin was 1.2 mmol/l. After a median follow-up of 3.9 years, there were 83 events in the atorvastatin group and 127 in the placebo group (risk reduction in first major cardiovascular events: 37%; 95% CI: -52 to -17; p = 0.001). The study was not powered on overall mortality but there were 82 deaths in the placebo group compared with 61 in the treatment group (risk reduction: 27%; HR 0.73; 95% CI: 0.52 to 1.01; p = 0.059). In CARDS, allocation of 1,000 patients to atorvastatin therapy would avoid 37 first major CVD events over a 4-year follow-up and 27 patients would need to be treated for 4 years to prevent one event. If first and subsequent events are included, 50 major CVD events would be prevented over a 4-year follow-up period.[28]

Subsequent pre-planned analyses of the CARDS database have demonstrated that the benefit of atorvastatin occurred early in the trial and was statistically significant at 18 months.[29] It is clear that the elderly (>65 years) benefit to the same extent as younger patients with, importantly, no increase in side effects.[30] Indeed, in CARDS, there was no overall difference in clinical or biochemical adverse events between the placebo and treated groups. A cost-benefit analysis has demonstrated that the intervention was cost-effective, even for those at lower risk, as assessed by the UKPDS risk engine.[31]

The clinical implications from CARDS are wide-ranging. At baseline, two-thirds of patients had LDL cholesterol levels <3.35 mmol/dl (130 mg/dl) which correspond to the previous unequivocal American Diabetes Association (ADA) treatment threshold of ≥3.35 mmol/dl. A quarter of patients had LDL cholesterol levels <2.6 mmol/l. Following treatment with atorvastatin, the median LDL cholesterol was 2 mmol/l and 75% achieved LDL cholesterol levels of 2.5 mmol/l or lower (25% had LDL cholesterol levels <1.7 mmol/l). The risk reduction observed in patients with baseline LDL cholesterol levels <3 mmol/l was statistically significant (p = 0.025). The risk reduction in patients (n = 743) with LDL cholesterol levels <2.6 mmol/l was 27%, but this effect did not achieve significance.[28] Therefore, CARDS demonstrated treatment benefits at levels of LDL cholesterol not previously recognised as requiring intervention. Indeed, it is clear from CARDS and HPS that it is the level of risk that should be the major determinant of statin therapy rather than the LDL cholesterol level.

LDL cholesterol lowering and stroke

Cerebrovascular disease represents a significant health burden and 10% of all deaths in developed countries are due to stroke.[32] At 6 months, of ischaemic stroke survivors aged

≥65 years, residual hemiparesis is present in 50%, ambulatory problems in 31%, dependency in activities of daily living in 26%, aphasia in 19%, residency in nursing home in 26% and depressive symptoms in 35%.[33] The majority of strokes are ischaemic and diabetes increases the risk of stroke two- to four-fold in women and two- to three-fold in men.[34]

Although LDL cholesterol has not been recognised as a major risk factor for stroke, it became clear, from the early statin trials, that the incidence of stroke was reduced by statin therapy. In patients with established coronary disease, stroke was reduced by 30% in 4S, 31% in CARE, 19% in LIPID, 25% in HPS, 25% in TNT and 13% in IDEAL for those in the treatment arm compared with the control arm.[15–17,35] In a meta-analysis of 26 statin trials, stroke was reduced by 21% (p<0.0001) in the treatment arm compared with control.[36] In this analysis it was estimated that each 10% reduction in LDL cholesterol was associated with a reduction in stroke risk of 15.6%.[36] In the meta-analysis of the four trials that compared more intensive statin therapy with conventional therapy, stroke was reduced by a further 18%.[26] In patients without previous CVD, stroke was reduced by 11% in West of Scotland Coronary Prevention Study (WOSCOPS),[37] 26% in HPS,[17,18] 27% in ASCOT–LLA[27] and 48% in CARDS.[28] The results of ASCOT–LLA are particularly interesting as they were observed in a population with hypertension that was well-treated.[27]

Of note, the only information in relation to subsequent stroke risk in patients with previous cerebrovascular disease came from HPS.[17] In the group allocated to simvastatin 40 mg/day, there were 169 subsequent strokes compared with 170 in the placebo group, indicating no effect of the drug. Recently, the results of the Stroke Prevention by Aggressive Reduction in Cholesterol Levels (SPARCL) trial have demonstrated, for the first time in a specific population with previous stroke, that intensive LDL cholesterol lowering with atorvastatin 80 mg/day was associated with a 16% reduction in subsequent stroke, together with large benefits in CHD reduction compared with placebo.[38] Analysis of the diabetic subgroup from this trial is eagerly awaited.

Conclusion

In this short article I have highlighted some of the evidence from RCTs using statins which inform clinical care of patients with diabetes, particularly the more recent trials which indicate that more clinical benefit can be obtained if LDL cholesterol concentrations are more intensively lowered. On the basis of these trials, important national and international bodies have suggested that goals for LDL cholesterol should be tightened. The JBS2 guidelines have also provided new guidance that the LDL cholesterol goal should be 2 mmol/l. In this author's opinion, this is entirely reasonable in the population with diabetes given the high residual risk of CVD events, particularly in patients with established CVD. The guidelines from JBS2 for diabetes are shown in Table 2.

Table 2: The JBS2 guidelines on prevention of cardiovascular disease in clinical practice.[3]

Indications for statin therapy in diabetes	Targets

• Aged >40 yrs type 2 or type 1
 • Aged 18–39 yrs type 2 or type 1 and
   – Significant retinopathy
   – Nephropathy
   – Poor glycaemic control (HbA$_{1c}$>9%)
   – Hypertension
   – Cholesterol >6 mmol/l
   – Features of metabolic syndrome:
     Triglyceride >1.7 mmol/l; HDL <1.0
     in men, <1.2 mmol/l in women
   – Family history of premature CVD
     in first degree relative
	Total cholesterol <4 mmol/l
	 LDL-cholesterol <2 mmol/l

It is the duty of physicians trusted with the care of this high-risk population to apply these new guidelines to their everyday care of patients so that the huge toll of macrovascular disease can be reduced. I commend them to you.

References

1. Zimmet PZ, Alberti KGMM. The changing face of macrovascular disease in non-insulin-dependent diabetes mellitus: an epidemic in progress. *Lancet* 1997; **350** (Suppl 1): 1–4.

2. Betteridge DJ. Dyslipidaemia and diabetes. *Pract Diabetes Int* 2001; **18**: 201–8.

3. JBS 2 Joint British Societies' guidelines on prevention of cardiovascular disease in clinical practice. *Heart* 2005; **91**: Suppl V.

4. British Cardiac Society, British Hyperlipidaemia Association, British Hypertension Society, British Diabetic Association. Joint British recommendations on prevention of coronary heart disease in clinical practice: summary. *BMJ* 2000; **320**: 705–8.

5. Taskinen MR. Diabetic dyslipidaemia: from basic research to clinical practice. *Diabetologia* 2003: **46**: 733–49.

6. Stamler J, Vaccaro O, Neaton JD, *et al*. Diabetes, other risk factors and 12 year cardiovascular mortality for men screened in the Multiple Risk Factor Intervention Trial. *Diabetes Care* 1993; **16**: 434–44.

7. Turner RC, Millns H, Neil HAW *et al*. Risk factors for coronary artery disease in non-insulin dependent diabetes mellitus: United Kingdom Prospective Diabetes Study (UKPDS: 23). *BMJ* 1998; **316**: 823–8.

8. Chapman MJ, Guerin M, Bruckert E. Atherogenic dense low density lipoproteins: pathophysiology and new therapeutic approaches. *Eur Heart J* 1998: **19**: (Suppl A) A24–A30.

9. Chait A, Wight TN. Interaction of native and modified low density lipoproteins with extracellular matrix. *Curr Opin Lipidol* 2000; **11**: 451–6.

10. Sniderman AD, Scantlebury T, Cianflone K. Hypertriglyceridaemic hyper apoB: the unappreciated atherogenic dyslipidaemia in type 2 diabetes mellitus. *Ann Intern Med* 2001; **135**: 447–59.

11. Betteridge DJ, Khan M. In: *Statins and Coronary Artery Disease* (2nd edn). London: Science Press, 2003.

12. The Scandinavian Simvastatin Survival Study Group. Randomised trial of cholesterol lowering in 4444 people with coronary heart disease: the Scandinavian simvastatin survival study (4S). *Lancet* 1994; **344**: 1383–9.

13. Pyörälä K, Pedersen TR, Kjekshus J *et al*. Cholesterol lowering with simvastatin improves prognosis of diabetic patients with coronary heart disease. A subgroup analysis of the Scandinavian Simvastatin Survival Study (4S). *Diabetes Care* 1997; **20**: 614–20.

14. Haffner SM, Alexander CM, Cook TJ *et al*. Reduced coronary events in simvastatin-treated patients with coronary heart disease and diabetes or impaired fasting glucose levels. Subgroup analysis in the Scandinavian Simvastatin Survival Study. *Arch Int Med* 1999; **159**: 2661–7.

15. Lewis SJ, Moye LA, Sacks FM *et al*. Effect of pravastatin on cardiovascular events in older people with MI and cholesterol levels in the average range. Results of the cholesterol and recurrent events trial (CARE) trial. *Ann Intern Med* 1998; **129**: 681–9.

16. The Long-Term Intervention with Pravastatin in Ischaemic Disease (LIPID) Study Group. Prevention of cardiovascular events and death with pravastatin in people with coronary heart disease and a broad range of initial cholesterol levels. The long-term intervention with pravastatin in ischaemic disease (LIPID) study. *N Engl J Med* 1998; **339**: 1349–57.

17. Heart Protection Study Collaborative Group. MRC/BHF heart protection study of cholesterol lowering with simvastatin in 20,536 high risk individuals: a randomised placebo-controlled trial. *Lancet* 2002; **360**: 7–22.

18. Heart Protection Study Collaborative Group. MRC/BHF Heart Protection Study of cholesterol lowering with simvastatin in 5963 people with diabetes: a randomized placebo-controlled trial. *Lancet* 2003; **361**: 2005–16.

19. Cholesterol Treatment Trialists' (CTT) Collaborators. Efficacy and safety of cholesterol-lowering treatment: prospective meta-analysis of data from 90,056 participants in 14 randomised trials of statins. *Lancet* 2005; **366**: 1267–78.

20. Cannon CP, Braunwald E, Mccabe CH *et al*. Intensive versus moderate lipid-lowering with statins after acute coronary syndromes. *N Engl J Med* 2004; **350**: 1495–504.

21. Ahmed S, Cannon CP, Murphy SA, Braunwald E. Acute coronary syndromes and diabetes: is intensive lipid lowering beneficial? Results of the PROVE IT-TIMI 22 trial. *Eur Heart J* 2006; **27**: 2323–9.

22. LaRosa JC, Grundy SM, Waters D *et al*. Intensive lipid lowering with atorvastatin in patients with stable coronary disease. *N Engl J Med* 2005; **352**: 1425–35.

23. Shepherd J, Barter P, Carmena R *et al*. Effect of lowering LDL cholesterol substantially below recommended levels in patients with coronary heart disease: the Treating to New Targets (TNT) Study. *Diabetes Care* 2006; **29**: 1220–6.

24. Grundy SM, Cleeman JI, Merz CNB *et al*. Implications of recent clinical trials for the National Cholesterol Education Program Adult Treatment Panel III Guidelines. *Circulation* 2004; **110**: 227–39.

25. The Task Force on Diabetes and Cardiovascular Diseases of the European Society of Cardiology (ESC) and of the European Association for the Study of Diabetes (EASD). Ryden L, Standl E, Bartnik M *et al*. Guidelines on diabetes, pre-diabetes and cardiovascular diseases: executive summary. *Eur Heart J* 2007; **28**: 88–136.

26. Cannon CP, Steinberg BA, Murphy SA *et al*. Meta-analysis of cardiovascular outcomes trials comparing intensive versus moderate statin therapy. *JACC* 2006; **48**: 438–55.

27. Sever PS, Dahlof B, Poylter NR *et al*. Prevention of coronary and strokes events with atorvastatin in hypertensive patients who have average or lower than average cholesterol concentrations in the Anglo-Scandinavian Cardiac Outcomes Trial-Lipid Lowering Arm (ASCOT–LLA): a multicentre randomized controlled study. *Lancet* 2003; **361**: 1149–58.

28. Colhoun HM, Betteridge DJ, Durrington PN *et al*. Primary prevention of cardiovascular disease in type 2 diabetes in the Collaborative Atorvastatin Diabetes Study (CARDS): multicentre randomized placebo-controlled trial. *Lancet* 2004; **364**: 685–96.

29. Colhoun HM, Betteridge DJ, Durrington PN *et al*. Rapid emergence of effect of atorvastatin on cardiovascular outcomes in the Collaborative Atorvastatin Diabetes Study (CARDS). *Diabetologia* 2005; **48**: 2482–85.

30. Neil HA, DeMicco DA, Luo D *et al*. Analysis of efficacy and safety in patients aged 65–75 years at randomization: Collaborative Atorvastatin Diabetes Study (CARDS). *Diabetes Care* 2006; **29**: 2378–84.

31. Raikou M, McGuire A, Colhoun HM *et al*. Cost-effectiveness of primary prevention of cardiovascular disease with atorvastatin in type 2 diabetes: results from the Collaborative Atorvastatin Diabetes Study (CARDS). *Diabetologia* 2007; **50**: 733–40.

32. Rothwell PM, Coull AJ, Silver LE *et al*. Population-based study of event-rate, incidence, case fatality, and mortality for all acute vascular events in all arterial territories. (Oxford Vascular Study) *Lancet* 2005; **366**: 1773–83.

33. Kelly-Hayes M, Beiser A, Kase CS *et al*. The influence of gender and age on disability following ischaemic stroke: the Framingham Study. *J Stroke Cerebrovasc Dis* 2003; **12**: 119–26.

34. Almdal T, Scharling H, Jan Skov Jensen JS, Vestergaard H. The independent effect of type 2 diabetes mellitus on ischemic heart disease, stroke, and death: A population-based study of 13,000 men and women with 20 years of follow-up. *Arch Intern Med* 2004; **164**: 1422–6.

35. Pedersen TR, Faergeman O, Kastelein JJP *et al*. High-dose atorvastatin vs usual-dose simvastatin for secondary prevention after myocardial infarction. The IDEAL Study; a randomized controlled trial. *JAMA* 2005; **294**: 2437–45.

36. Amarenco P, Labreuche J, Lavallée P, Touboul P-J. Statins in stroke prevention and carotid atherosclerosis: systematic review and up-to-date meta-analysis. *Stroke* 2004 **35**: 2902–9.

37. Shepherd J, Cobbe SM, Ford I *et al*. Prevention of coronary heart disease with pravastatin in men with hypercholesterolaemia. *N Engl J Med* 1995; **333**: 1301–7.

38. The Stroke Prevention by Aggressive Reduction in Cholesterol Levels (SPARCL) Investigators. High-dose atorvastatin after stroke or transient ischaemic attack. *N Engl J Med* 2006; **355**: 549–59.

Diabetogenicity of antihypertensive therapy

Dr Ajay K Gupta and Professor Neil R Poulter

Key points

- Antihypertensive therapy, particularly beta-blockers and diuretics, variably influences the propensity of hypertensive patients to develop new-onset diabetes (NOD).
- The risk of associated NOD is increased by the use of β-blockers and diuretics and reduced with angiotensin-receptor blockers and angiotensin-converting enzyme inhibitors with calcium-channel blockers being neutral.
- Increased levels of fasting plasma glucose, body mass index, serum triglyceride and systolic blood pressure are among other significant risk factors for NOD in hypertensive patients.
- Whilst controversy persists regarding the impact of antihypertensive-associated incident diabetes on cardiovascular disease, optimal antihypertensive therapy should not induce a major diabetogenic effect.

Introduction

Both hypertension and type 2 diabetes are significant risk factors for cardiovascular disease (CVD), and frequently co-exist, with a complex inter-relationship. Compared with normotensive people, patients with hypertension have a 2–3-times greater risk of developing new-onset diabetes (NOD).[1] Several studies have shown that this increased propensity of hypertensive patients to develop NOD is variably influenced by antihypertensive drugs – particularly β-blockers and diuretics.[1-4] However, globally, these drugs continue to be among the most commonly used antihypertensive agents. This is in part due to the reported findings of a number of studies which, despite showing adverse metabolic effects, including increased rates of NOD associated with the use of these drugs, have failed to demonstrate any associated increase in adverse cardiovascular outcomes.[5,6] These findings have been interpreted as adding some credence to the claim that drug-induced diabetes is 'innocent'.[7] However this message is counter-intuitive and other studies have shown an increased cardiovascular toll associated with incident diabetes[8] or increased fasting serum glucose associated with the use of antihypertensive drugs.[9] We herein review evidence relating to the diabetogenicity of various antihypertensive agents and the cardiovascular toll, if any, associated with incident diabetes.

Diabetogenic potential of antihypertensive agents

Even though the adverse metabolic effects of diuretics and β-blockers, particularly impairment of glucose tolerance and worsening of lipid profiles, have been known since the mid-1960s,[10–12] their extrapolation into an increased incidence of diabetes was not properly acknowledged until the publication of observational studies in the mid-1990s.[1,13–16] In an observational study of 12,550 hypertensive patients without diabetes at baseline, a 28% greater risk of NOD was observed with the use of β-blockers (relative hazard 1.28; 95% confidence interval (CI): 1.04–1.57).[1] In contrast, the use of other antihypertensive agents, such as angiotensin-converting enzyme (ACE) inhibitors, diuretics and calcium-channel blockers (CCBs), was not associated with any significant difference in incidence of NOD compared with those who were not taking any antihypertensive medications. Interestingly, although use of diuretics was not associated with an increased risk of NOD,[1] it was associated with a significant increase in fasting serum glucose in the first 3 years of observation. In another retrospective, population-based cohort study based on prescriptions of antihypertensive drugs as an exposure among 76,176 elderly people with hypertension aged ≥66 years, no difference was observed in the incidence of diabetes among the users of β-blockers, ACE inhibitors and CCBs.[17] More recently, in an analysis of three, large, prospective cohorts (Nurses Health Study (NHS) I & II, and the Health Professionals Follow-up Study (HPFS)), 3,589 cases of incident diabetes were observed among the 41,993 older women (NHS I), 14,151 younger women (NHS II) and 19,472 men (HPFS) with a history of hypertension.[18] On multivariate analysis, adjusting for age, BMI and physical activity, the use of β-blockers compared with those not taking β-blockers, was associated with a significantly increased risk of NOD among both older women (32%; 95% CI: 1.20–1.46) and men (20%; 95% CI: 1.05–1.38). Similarly, the use of thiazides, compared with patients not taking a thiazide, was independently associated with increased risks of 20%, 45% and 36% among older women, younger women and men, respectively.

All of these studies, being observational, have been criticised because of small sample size,[14,16] lack of statistical power, inadequate adjustment for confounders,[13,16–18] inappropriate reference group, self-reported ascertainment,[18] selection bias[16] and short follow-up.[17]

NOD in randomised, clinical trials in patients with hypertension

Over the last decade or so, a number of trials have reported on incident diabetes (Figure 1).[19]

Most of these trials have compared the efficacy of older, 'standard' antihypertensive agents (β-blockers, diuretics, or their combination) with newer antihypertensive agents (CCBs, ACE inhibitors and angiotensin-receptor blockers (ARBs)). However a few trials, mainly in patients without hypertension, have also compared the incidence of NOD

Figure 1: Incidence of new diabetes according to study and drug treatment.[19]

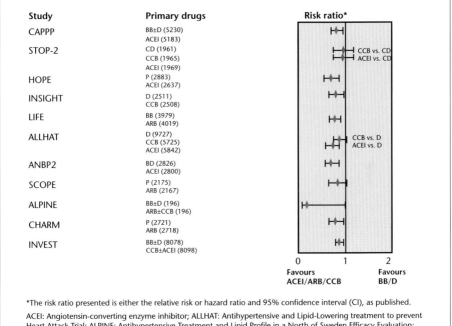

*The risk ratio presented is either the relative risk or hazard ratio and 95% confidence interval (CI), as published.

ACEI: Angiotensin-converting enzyme inhibitor; ALLHAT: Antihypertensive and Lipid-Lowering treatment to prevent Heart Attack Trial; ALPINE: Antihypertensive Treatment and Lipid Profile in a North of Sweden Efficacy Evaluation; ANBP2: Second Australian National Blood Pressure Study; ARB: Angiotensin II receptor blocker; BB: β-blocker; CAPPP: Captopril Prevention Project; CCB: Calcium channel blocker; CD: Conventional drugs; CHARM: Candesartan in Heart failure Assessment of Reduction in Mortality and Morbidity; D: Diuretic; INSIGHT: Intervention as a Goal in Hypertension Treatment; INVEST: International Verapamil-Trandolapril Study; LIFE: Losartan Intervention For Endpoint reduction; P: Placebo

using an active drug with placebo. These studies consistently favour use of the newer, metabolically neutral therapies (ACE inhibitors, ARBs or CCBs). In these trials, the average risk reduction compared with conventional therapy was 20% for ACE inhibitors or ARBs (p <0.001) and 16% for CCBs (p <0.001).[20] However, there are methodological issues pertaining to some of these studies. For example, in the Antihypertensive and Lipid-Lowering Treatment to Prevent Heart Attack Trial (ALLHAT) and Heart Outcomes Prevention Evaluation (HOPE) study, NOD was not considered as an end-point *a priori*. Follow-up was incomplete in some trials, such as ALLHAT, in which only 38% of the patients had fasting plasma glucose (FPG) values measured at the end of 4 years.[4] In other trials, there were issues related to the definition of NOD, and contamination of results by use of β-blockers or diuretics in both arms. A number of studies were too small to give adequate statistical power, whilst others used an open-labelled, blinded end-point design, thereby increasing the likelihood of detection bias.

Recently, the results of the Anglo–Scandinavian Cardiac Outcomes Trial – Blood Pressure Lowering Arm (ASCOT–BPLA),[21] of which NOD was one of the pre-specified outcomes, showed that an amlodipine-based regimen (amlodipine ± perindopril) compared with an atenolol-based regimen (atenolol ± thiazide) was associated with reduced risk of NOD of about one third (Figure 2).

Figure 2: New-onset diabetes* in ASCOT-BPLA.[21]

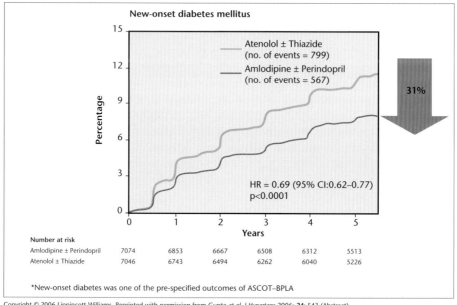

However, in this trial, like most others, it is difficult to clarify whether the differences in NOD between the two treatment arms were due to the diabetogenicity of the β-blocker/diuretic combination, or protection afforded by the use of the ACE inhibitor, which was added to amlodipine. Nevertheless, results from studies such as the Valsartan Antihypertensive Long-term Use Evaluation (VALUE) trial, comparing the CCB, amlodipine with the ARB, valsartan, and other placebo-controlled trials using ACE inhibitors, ARBs and diuretics, suggest that the bulk of the difference could be due to the diabetogenicity of β-blockers and diuretics, with some protection afforded by the ACE inhibitor and the CCB being metabolically neutral.

Most recently, part of the Diabetes REduction Assessment with ramipril and rosiglitazone Medication (DREAM) trial compared ramipril with placebo in relation to the primary outcome of a composite of death and NOD among patients with impaired glycaemia but without any previous cardiovascular events.[22] During a median follow-up of 3 years, use of ramipril 15 mg once-daily did not produce significant protection against NOD. However, the results suggested a protective effect (hazard ratio

(HR) 0.91; 95% CI: 0.81–1.03; p = 0.15) and there was a significant improvement in reversal of impaired glycaemia with a reduction in glucose levels at 2 hours post-glucose load in the ramipril group (p = 0.01). These findings are compatible with other data suggesting that ACE inhibitors do have a beneficial effect on impaired glycaemia. That these effects were less than expected in the DREAM trial may reflect the low cardiovascular risk of the patients recruited and the limited power to detect significant differences in NOD in such a short duration of follow-up.

In summary, most trials of antihypertensive agents attest to the presence of differences in diabetogenicity of various antihypertensive agents. However, due to the heterogeneity amongst these trials, drug classes are often difficult to compare, even in meta-analysis. Recently, results of a network meta-analysis – a 'controversial' statistical technique to allow direct and indirect comparison of different treatment strategies – have allowed comparisons among different classes of antihypertensive agents despite the heterogeneity of the trials involved.[3] In this analysis, data from 22 clinical trials comprising 143,153 participants without diabetes at randomisation were analysed in relation to NOD. The results suggest that the association between antihypertensive agents and incident diabetes is lowest for ARB and ACE inhibitors, followed by CCB and placebo, with β-blockers and diuretics increasing the risk. Figure 3 illustrates this relative ranking of different antihypertensive classes using initial use of diuretic therapy as a reference group.

Figure 3: Results of network meta-analysis of 22 clinical trials showing the incidence of NOD with different anti-hypertensive agents.[3]

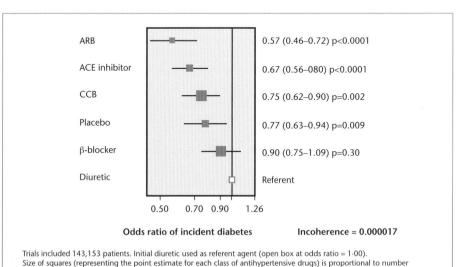

Trials included 143,153 patients. Initial diuretic used as referent agent (open box at odds ratio = 1·00). Size of squares (representing the point estimate for each class of antihypertensive drugs) is proportional to number of patients who developed incident diabetes. Horizontal lines indicate 95% CI. Odds ratios to the left of the vertical line at unity denote a protective effect (compared with initial diuretic). Individual pair-wise comparisons between diuretic vs β-blocker (p = 0·30), placebo vs CCB (0·72), ACE inhibitor vs ARB (0·16) did not achieve significance (p <0·05).

The rank order remains the same even if placebo is used as a reference group. However, in this situation, only the initial use of ARB (odds ratio (OR) 0.75; 95% CI: 0.61–0.91) and diuretic therapy (OR 1.3; 95% CI: 1.07–1.58) retain significance, whilst ACE inhibitors (OR: 0.87; 95% CI: 0.75–1.01), CCBs (OR: 0.97; 95% CI: 0.82–1.15) and β-blockers (OR: 1.17; 95% CI: 0.98–1.40) were non-significantly different from placebo. Interestingly, the beneficial, albeit non-significant, effect of ACE inhibitors in comparison to placebo is similar to that observed in the DREAM trial.

Predictors of NOD in patients with hypertension

The above studies have established the role of antihypertensive therapy – particularly β-blockers and diuretics – in influencing the propensity of subjects with hypertension to develop incident diabetes. However, little is known about the other baseline predictors of NOD and the importance of antihypertensive therapy relative to these variables. FPG and body mass index (BMI) were found to be important determinants in earlier trials.[23,24] In ASCOT–BPLA, on multivariable analysis of 14,120 hypertensive patients without diabetes at baseline,[21] higher levels of FPG, BMI, serum triglyceride and systolic blood pressure were found to be the major significant risk factors for NOD. In contrast, amlodipine-based treatment (HR 0.66; 95% CI: 0.59–0.74), high, high-density lipoprotein (HDL) cholesterol, alcohol use, total cholesterol and age >55 years were found to be significantly protective factors. In this trial, as in others, FPG was the most powerful predictor with risk increasing 5.8-fold (95% CI: 5.23–6.43) for each 1 mmol/l rise above 5 mmol/l. Risk increased by 49% for each 5-unit increase in BMI (up to 35 kg/m^2) and by 12% for each 1 mmol/l increase in serum triglyceride levels. In contrast, randomisation to amlodipine-based treatment and increase in baseline HDL by 1 mmol/l reduced the risk by 34% and 28%, respectively.

Since most of these baseline predictors are modifiable by pharmacotherapy and/or life-style modification, it is conceivable that better management during follow-up may also prevent incident diabetes. However, at present, the impact of changes in these predictors during follow-up, on development of NOD, is unknown.

Incident diabetes: innocent or malign?

Several studies have evaluated the effect of antihypertensive-associated incident diabetes and/or dysglycaemia on cardiovascular mortality and morbidity, often with conflicting results.[5,6,8,9] Kostis et al., in their 14.3-year follow-up of the Systolic Hypertension in the Elderly Program (SHEP), reported that even though the diuretic therapy (as compared with placebo) was associated with increased risk of NOD, the cardiovascular mortality in those who developed incident diabetes while on diuretic treatment (HR 1.04; 95% CI: 0.74–1.45) was insignificant and much less then those who developed incident diabetes while on placebo (HR 1.56; 95% CI: 1.17–2.18).[5]

In contrast, those with diabetes at baseline, regardless of the treatment group, had significantly increased risk of cardiovascular mortality (HR 1.66; 95% CI: 1.41–1.95) (Figure 4).

Figure 4: Type 2 diabetes (A) and NOD (B): Kaplan–Meier curves of cardiovascular mortality and all-cause mortality outcomes in SHEP after 14.3 years of median follow-up.[5]

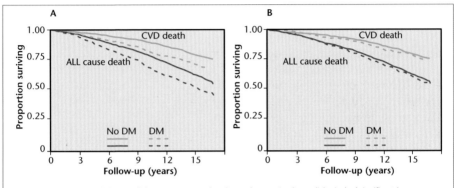

Patients with previously known diabetes, as compared to those who remained non-diabetic, had significant increases in cardiovascular and all-cause mortality (A). In contrast, those with incident diabetes, as compared to those without diabetes, were not found to be associated with a significant increase in either cardiovascular or all cause mortality (B).

Based on these observational findings, the authors concluded that diuretic-associated NOD runs a much milder course, and has no significant increase in adverse cardiovascular risk. However, these results can be explained on the basis of the favourable blood pressure difference of 11.3/3.4 mmHg that was observed in patients on diuretic therapy. Since blood pressure control in patients with diabetes is one of the most important factors in the prevention of CVD,[25] it seems likely that the incremental cardiovascular risk associated with a few incident cases of diabetes in the diuretic arm of SHEP would be more than compensated for by the considerable reduction in cardiovascular risk caused by the large blood-pressure reduction induced by the diuretic. More recently, a *post-hoc* analysis of the ALLHAT trial also suggested that diuretic-associated incident diabetes may be 'innocent'.[6,7] Although this was a large trial, there were several methodological shortcomings in these analyses. For example, only 53% of the analysed patients had one or more FPG levels recorded at any time during follow-up, misclassification of diabetic patients into the non-diabetic group was common, and the definition of NOD used was inadequate (single reading of FPG >125 mg/dl (6.9 mmol/l)).[26]

In contrast to the findings described above, a small number of studies have shown an increased cardiovascular toll associated with incident diabetes[8] or increased FPG associated with antihypertensive drugs.[9] Verdecchia *et al.* in their small cohort study of 795 initially untreated, hypertensive patients followed-up for a median of 6 years, observed NOD in approximately 6%.[8] They reported that antihypertensive-associated incident diabetes was associated with an almost three-fold increased risk of CVD when compared with patients persistently free from diabetes. The event rates in patients with antihypertensive-associated incident diabetes were similar to those who had diabetes at baseline (Figure 5).

Figure 5: Hypertensive patients with new-onset diabetes have similar cardiovascular risk as patients with existing diabetes.*[8]

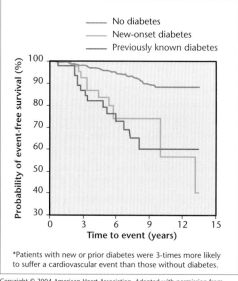

— No diabetes
— New-onset diabetes
— Previously known diabetes

*Patients with new or prior diabetes were 3-times more likely to suffer a cardiovascular event than those without diabetes.

Copyright © 2004 American Heart Association. Adapted with permission from Verdecchia *et al. Hypertension* 2004; **43**: 963–9.

Similarly, Dunder *et al.*, in their observational study of 1,860 men, reported that increase in blood glucose was an independent risk factor for myocardial infarction in men receiving antihypertensive agents (mainly β-blockers and diuretics), but not in those without.[9] However, all of these studies have been appropriately criticised for the small number of NOD cases which ultimately limit their power.

These apparently conflicting results notwithstanding, we hypothesize that the analytical approach in these trials, using development of NOD as a dichotomous point of abrupt increased risk, do not take into account the increased cardiovascular risk associated with impaired glucose regulation and β-cell dysfunction, which may in fact occur up to a decade before the diagnosis of NOD is made. Several observational studies have shown a continuous graded relationship between cardiovascular risk across the whole range of glucose levels.[1,27] Thus, comparing event rates among patients with and without NOD, even when numbers were larger, is to obscure real differences in rates between truly dysglycaemic and normoglycaemic individuals.

Conclusion

In summary, the diabetogenic potential of antihypertensive agents such as β-blockers and diuretics is now established. However, doubt remains about the extent of the size of the protection afforded by use of ARBs and ACE inhibitors against the development of NOD. It has yet to be established conclusively whether the diabetogenicity associated with antihypertensive agents manifests itself as adverse cardiovascular outcomes. However, pending newer and more robust evidence, it seems reasonable to try to avoid diabetogenic agents, and therefore unwise not to use metabolically neutral or beneficial antihypertensive agents, particularly since these agents have been shown to be more cost-effective.[28]

References

1. Gress TW, Nieto FJ, Shahar E *et al.* Hypertension and antihypertensive therapy as risk factors for type 2 diabetes mellitus. *N Engl J Med* 2000; **342**: 905–12.

2. Mancia G, Grassi G, Zanchetti A. New-onset diabetes and antihypertensive drugs. *J Hypertens* 2006; **24**: 3–10.

3. Elliott WJ, Meyer PM. Incident diabetes in clinical trials of antihypertensive drugs: a network meta-analysis. *Lancet* 2007; **369**: 201–7.

4. Padwal R, Majumdar SR, Johnson JA *et al.* A systematic review of drug therapy to delay or prevent type 2 diabetes. *Diabetes Care* 2005; **28**: 736–44.

5. Kostis JB, Wilson AC, Freudenberger RS *et al.* Long-term effect of diuretic-based therapy on fatal outcomes in subjects with isolated systolic hypertension with and without diabetes. *Am J Cardiol* 2005; **95**: 29–35.

6. Barzilay JI, Davis BR, Cutler JA *et al.* Fasting glucose levels and incident diabetes mellitus in older nondiabetic adults randomized to receive 3 different classes of antihypertensive treatment: a report from the Antihypertensive and Lipid-Lowering Treatment to Prevent Heart Attack Trial (ALLHAT). *Arch Intern Med* 2006; **166**: 2191–201.

7. Phillips RA. New-onset diabetes mellitus less deadly than elevated blood pressure? Following the evidence in the administration of thiazide diuretics. *Arch Intern Med* 2006; **166**: 2174–6.

8. Verdecchia P, Reboldi G, Angeli F *et al.* Adverse prognostic significance of new diabetes in treated hypertensive subjects. *Hypertension* 2004; **43**: 963–9.

9. Dunder K, Lind L, Zethelius B *et al.* Increase in blood glucose concentration during antihypertensive treatment as a predictor of myocardial infarction: population based cohort study. *Br Med J* 2003; **326**: 681.

10. Goldner MG, Zarowitz H, Akgun S. Hyperglycemia and glycosuria due to thiazide derivatives administered in diabetes mellitus. *N Engl J Med* 1960; **262**: 403–5.

11. Furman BL. Impairment of glucose tolerance produced by diuretics and other drugs. *Pharmacol Ther* 1981; **12**: 613–49.

12. Houston MC. Adverse effects of antihypertensive drug therapy on glucose intolerance. *Cardiol Clin* 1986; **4**: 117–35.

13. Mykkänen L, Kuusisto J, Pyörälä K *et al.* Increased risk of non-insulin-dependent diabetes mellitus in elderly hypertensive subjects. *J Hypertens* 1994; **12**: 1425–32.

14. Samuelsson O, Hedner T, Berglund G *et al.* Diabetes mellitus in treated hypertension: incidence, predictive factors and the impact of non-selective beta-blockers and thiazide diuretics during 15 years treatment of middle-aged hypertensive men in the Primary Prevention Trial Goteborg, Sweden. *J Hum Hypertens* 1994; **8**: 257–63.

15. Skarfors ET, Selinus KI, Lithell HO. Risk factors for developing non-insulin dependent diabetes: a 10-year follow up of men in Uppsala. *Br Med J* 1991; **303**: 755–60.

16. Rajala U, Qiao Q, Laakso M, Keinanen-Kiukaanniemi S. Antihypertensive drugs as predictors of type 2 diabetes among subjects with impaired glucose tolerance. *Diabetes Res Clin Pract* 2000; **50**: 231–9.

17. Padwal R, Mamdani M, Alter DA *et al.* Antihypertensive therapy and incidence of type 2 diabetes in an elderly cohort. *Diabetes Care* 2004; **27**: 2458–63.

18. Taylor EN, Hu FB, Curhan GC. Antihypertensive medications and the risk of incident type 2 diabetes. *Diabetes Care* 2006; **29**: 1065–70.

19. Pepine CJ, Cooper-Dehoff RM. Cardiovascular therapies and risk for development of diabetes. *J Am Coll Cardiol* 2004; **44**: 509–12.

20. Opie LH, Schall R. Old antihypertensives and new diabetes. *J Hypertens* 2004; **22**: 1453–8.

21. Gupta A, Poulter NR, Dahlof B *et al.* Determinants of new onset diabetes among hypertensive patients randomised in ASCOT–BPLA (Abstract). *Journal of Hypertension* 2006; **24** (Suppl): S43.

22. Bosch J, Yusuf S, Gerstein HC *et al.* Effect of ramipril on the incidence of diabetes. *N Engl J Med* 2006; **355**: 1551–62.

23. Niklason A, Hedner T, Niskanen L, Lanke J. Development of diabetes is retarded by ACE inhibition in hypertensive patients – a subanalysis of the Captopril Prevention Project (CAPPP). *J Hypertens* 2004; **22**: 645–52.

24. Lindholm LH, Ibsen H, Borch-Johnsen K *et al.* Risk of new-onset diabetes in the Losartan Intervention For Endpoint reduction in hypertension study. *J Hypertens* 2002; **20**: 1879–86.

25. UKPDS. Tight blood pressure control and risk of macrovascular and microvascular complications in type 2 diabetes: UKPDS 38. *BMJ* 1998; **317**: 703–13.

26. Gupta A, Poulter NR. Antihypertensive-associated incident diabetes: Controversy persists. *Arch Intern Med* 2007; **167**:1433.

27. Coutinho M, Gerstein HC, Wang Y, Yusuf S. The relationship between glucose and incident cardiovascular events. A meta-regression analysis of published data from 20 studies of 95,783 individuals followed for 12.4 years. *Diabetes Care* 1999; **22**: 233–40.

28. National Collaborating Centre for Chronic Conditions. Hypertension: management of hypertension in adults in primary care: partial update. *NICE Clinical Guideline.* London: Royal College of Physicians, 2006.

Diabetic retinopathy: medical management and screening

Dr Paul M Dodson

Key points

- Blindness in diabetic subjects is still all too common.
- The promising oral agents demonstrating benefit in human trials of patients with diabetic retinopathy are ruboxistaurin and fenofibrate.
- Ruboxistaurin has been shown to significantly reduce visual loss and laser requirement in patients with pre-proliferative retinopathy.
- Fenofibrate treatment has been demonstrated to significantly reduce laser treatment in type 2 diabetes over a 5-year period in the FIELD study.
- While the national screening programmes are being implemented, there is still debate on the exact level of quality assurance (QA) required, but recent experience does support the value of the English scheme QA protocol.
- The significance of only one or two micro-aneurysms in the retina (7.9% of patients with impaired glucose tolerance) has been suggested in the recent Diabetes Prevention Program study as indicative of diabetic retinopathy. This is in contrast to the findings in large studies of non-diabetic subjects in whom micro-aneurysms are found in 7.2%, thereby suggesting that this is not the case.

Medical management

Early in diabetes, intracellular hyperglycaemia causes abnormalities in blood flow and increased vascular permeability, reflecting the decreased activity of nitric oxide and increased activity of vasoconstrictors (e.g., angiotensin and endothelin-1), in addition to enhanced permeability factors [e.g., vascular endothelial growth factor (VEGF)].[1]

To date, there have been four main hypotheses of the causes of diabetic microvascular complications:
1. Increased polyol pathway flux
2. Increased advanced glycation end product formation
3. Activation of the protein kinase C (PKC) isoforms
4. Increased hexosamine pathway flux.[1]

Specific inhibitors of each of these pathways have been tested both *in vitro* and in animal models.[1]

Human trials of diabetic retinopathy (DR) have focused on the PKC inhibitors, growth factor inhibition (growth hormone and insulin-like growth factor-1), and the potential effects of lowering lipid levels. In particular, lipid lowering has become an area of considerable interest owing to the possibility of new, potential mechanisms and receptors where statins and fibrates may exert an effect.[2]

Two, large, randomised trials of growth hormone antagonism using somatostatin analogues have both recently reported an inconclusive result with no clear effect on the progression of pre-proliferative DR.[3] Previously, pilot studies had suggested that this therapeutic approach may also be beneficial in treating aggressive proliferative retinopathy, however, to date; this has not received any further investigation.

A role for angiotensin has been suggested in *in vitro* experiments and supported by the EURODIAB Controlled Trial of Lisinopril in Insulin-Dependent Diabetes (EUCLID) study in people with diabetes.[4] A large study of the potential benefit of an angiotensin-2 receptor blocker in both primary and secondary prevention of DR, the DIabetic Retinopathy Candesartan Trial (DIRECT), is currently underway.[5]

PKC inhibition

PKC is activated by hyperglycaemia-induced synthesis of diacyl glycerol I, resulting in increased VEGF levels and consequently, exudation from the retinal vessels. There are 12 isoforms of the PKC enzyme, but it is the PKC-β_2 isoform that is preferentially activated in the tissues involved in diabetic microvascular damage, particularly the retina.[2,6] Specific activation of PKC-β_2 increases retinal vascular permeability and neovascularisation in animal models.[2,6]

Ruboxistaurin

A novel drug, ruboxistaurin (proposed trade name Arxxant™, Eli Lilly & Co), which specifically blocks the PKC-β_2 isoform, has been identified. In animal studies, ruboxistaurin reduces retinal oedema and neovascularisation in diabetic animals, and antagonises the effects of VEGF when injected into the retinal circulation.[6] Initial results from clinical trials suggest a benefit in both diabetic macular oedema[7] and pre-proliferative retinopathy, with the latter showing reduced visual loss.[8] However, even though these trials suggested a clinical benefit, the primary endpoints did not reach statistical significance.[7,8]

The recent randomised, placebo-controlled, Phase III PKC β Inhibitor Diabetic Retinopathy Study (PKC–DRS2) has examined the potential of this new drug in 685 patients with diabetes, randomised to either placebo or 32 mg/day oral ruboxistaurin for a 3-year treatment period.[9] The mean patient age was 59 years and 88% had type 2 diabetes. The primary endpoint was the effect of ruboxistaurin on sustained moderate loss of vision in patients with moderately severe to very severe nonproliferative diabetic retinopathy, defined as 6 months of $\geq$15-letter loss on an Early Treatment of Diabetic Retinopathy Study (ETDRS) visual acuity (VA) chart.[9]

Results demonstrated a clinically and statistically significant decrease in visual loss (p<0.034) as well as a reduction in laser treatment, with most benefit in those with moderate to severe pre-proliferative retinopathy, with reduction of visual loss and progression of macular oedema (p<0.003) (Box 1).[9]

Box 1: Principal results from the PKC-DRS2.[9]

- Ruboxistaurin led to a 41% reduction in sustained visual loss (p = 0.01)
- There was a statistically significant 30% reduction in first application of laser (p = 0.018)
- Effects were apparent after 9–12 months of ruboxistaurin treatment
- Improvement in visual acuity (≥15 letters) with ruboxistaurin compared with placebo, 4.7 vs 2.4% (p = 0.021)
- Clinically significant macular oedema within 100 microns at baseline responded best: SMVL ruboxistaurin compared with placebo, 6.3 vs 12.1% (p = 0.033)
- Best response at ETDRS retinopathy level 53 of ruboxistaurin compared with placebo, 5.7 vs 12.6% (p = 0.014)
- Progression of DME from >100 microns to imminently vision-threatening stage of ruboxistaurin compared with placebo, 51.2 vs 64% (p = 0.047)
- Response to ruboxistaurin not exclusive to the presence of DME at baseline
- No change in progression of diabetic retinopathy ETDRS level between ruboxistaurin and placebo.

DME: Diabetic macular oedema; ETDRS: Early Treatment of Diabetic Retinopathy Study; SMVL: Sustained moderate visual loss.

Additionally, the safety profile of ruboxistaurin has shown no concerns and no real adverse effects, indeed, in this study the mortality rate was shown to be less in the ruboxistaurin group compared with placebo. Ruboxistaurin's licence application to the US Food and Drug Administration received an approvable letter requesting further Phase III data, and the manufacturer is currently deciding whether data can be obtained from existing trials, or whether a new study is required.[10] Conversely, no intravitreal anti-VEGF agent is currently licensed for use in the treatment of DR, despite being commonly used.

Lipid-lowering therapy

Statin and fibrate therapy have both been proven to reduce cardiovascular (CV) disease in patients with dyslipidaemia.[11] Older trials of lipid-lowering therapy carried out with clofibrate in exudative maculopathy have suggested that a reduction in macular exudates could be achieved with fibrates, but with little improvement in VA.[12,13] However the VA of patients examined in these trials were poor at the outset, and hence an improvement with lipid-lowering therapy was unrealistic.[11]

More recently, data have confirmed that increasing total cholesterol and low-density lipoprotein (LDL) levels, as well as increasing fasting serum triglycerides, is associated with a greater risk of developing maculopathy.[14] In addition, the Diabetes Control and Complications Trial (DCCT) group reported a similar relationship of increasing cholesterol levels with the development of macular oedema in patients with type 1 diabetes.[15] However, whilst these clinical studies do suggest a relationship between lipid-lowering and diabetic maculopathy, they do not prove causality or identify pathogenetic mechanisms.

Recent data have suggested a direct toxic effect of LDL on retinal capillary pericytes, and this effect can be enhanced by LDL glycation or oxidation.[16] A further *in vitro* study of human retinal endothelial cells also recently showed that the hypolipidaemic drug, fenofibrate, protected cells from apoptotic cell death as a result of serum deprivation through the sustained activation of the AMP-activated protein kinase (AMPK) pathway, and that it may influence VEGF mRNA expression.[17]

Thus, there is now compelling evidence that serum lipoproteins have a major role in exudative retinopathy in patients with diabetes, such that increasing total or LDL cholesterol is accepted as a risk factor for maculopathy. However, to date, there have been no large randomised trials to confirm a treatment effect with lipid lowering.

Small treatment trials with statins have, however, demonstrated benefit in the reduction of macular exudation and macular oedema.[11] The Collaborative Atorvastatin Diabetes Study (CARDS) assessed the effectiveness of atorvastatin 10 mg daily versus placebo for primary prevention of CV events in patients with type 2 diabetes.[18] Over 4 years, the results from CARDS demonstrated a trend to reduction of laser therapy undertaken in the atorvastatin arm (odds ratio 0.79, p = 0.14) (Figure 1), but no influence on diabetic retinopathy progression (author, personal communication). However, the interpretation of the latter is limited as the retinopathy status at study entry and endpoint was incomplete in half the patients.

Figure 1: Laser rates in the Collaborative Atorvastatin Diabetes Study (CARDS) (author, personal communication).

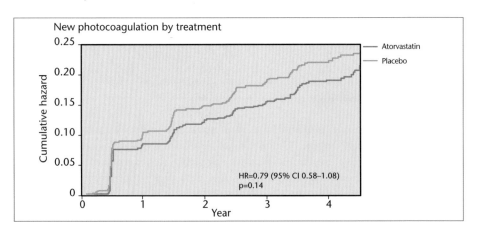

Likewise, the results of the Atorvastatin Study for Prevention of Coronary Heart Disease Endpoints in Non-Insulin-Dependent Diabetes Mellitus (ASPEN) study, studying the effects of atorvastatin on DR by photographic assessment, are awaited, along with those of a photographic sub-study of ASPEN. Thus the influence of statins on DR remains debated, but if there is an effect, it is likely to be small. It must also be acknowledged that the dosage of statins used in studies of DR so far have been low compared to the high dosages currently being prescribed (e.g., 40 mg simvastatin,

80 mg atorvastatin, and 20 mg rosuvastatin). It is hoped that the Action to Control CV Risk in Diabetes (ACCORD) Eye study (ACCORD-EYE) will provide further insight into the role of statins.[19]

The Fenofibrate Intervention and Event Lowering in Diabetes (FIELD) study, a large randomised trial designed to study the effects of fenofibrate 200 mg/day compared with placebo in the primary prevention of CV disease in type 2 diabetes, also included the evaluation of microvascular endpoints (Table 1).[20]

Table 1: The baseline characteristics of patients with type 2 diabetes entered into the FIELD study.[20]

	Placebo (n=1,900)	Fenofibrate (n=4,895)
Age at screening (mean years)	62	62
Current smoker (%)	9	9
Duration of diabetes (median, years)	5	5
HbA$_{1c}$ (median, %)	6.9	6.9
Hypertension (%)	56	57
– Systolic BP (mean mmHg)	141	140
– Diastolic BP (mean mmHg)	82	82

In this large, well conducted study, there was a highly significant reduction in laser eye treatment in patients previously untreated with laser (p<0.0004) (Figure 2).[20]

Figure 2: The reduction of laser endpoints in patients who were laser-naïve on entry to the FIELD trial.[20]

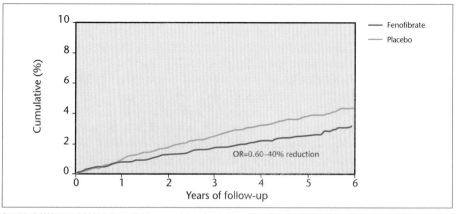

There was a 30% reduction in the number of patients needing one or more laser treatments for retinopathy in the fenofibrate group compared with placebo (p<0.0003).[20] This effect was achieved despite a significant increase in statin prescriptions in the placebo group (17%) compared with the fenofibrate group (8%, p<0.0001). Thus, it can be assumed that if statins did have an effect on DR, this would have resulted in a reduction in the treatment benefits observed with fenofibrate.

Ocular laser therapy is performed for a variety of different reasons, and includes yttrium aluminium garnet (YAG) laser for capsulotomy following cataract extraction, iridotomy for glaucoma treatment, and both panretinal and focal/grid laser for cases of retinal vein occlusion. Therefore, the nature of these laser endpoints needs to be determined. This is also true for other trials in DR such as the United Kingdom Prospective Diabetes Study (UKPDS) and CARDS. As a result, trial data do not yet prove the benefit of lipid lowering, and further data are awaited.

The ACCORD-EYE study, which is currently well underway, should allow further resolution of these issues.[19] The ACCORD-EYE study has been designed to assess the effects of the ACCORD medical treatment strategies of tight control of glycaemia and blood pressure and management of dyslipidaemia on the course of DR in patients with type 2 diabetes (n = 4,036). Specifically, it will address whether a treatment strategy using a fibrate and a statin reduces the development and progression of DR compared with one using placebo and a statin. It will also examine endpoints including loss of VA, cataract extraction and the development or progression of diabetic macular oedema.[19]

DR screening

Screening for the early signs of sight-threatening DR is worthwhile and cost effective, owing to the low cost of detection of retinopathy set against the large economic and social costs associated with blindness. Most importantly, laser treatment is most effective before the onset of visual symptoms, as it generally prevents visual loss (visual protection) rather than improving VA.[21]

The National DR Screening Programme[21] aims to provide systematic digital camera retinal screening through dilated pupils on an annual basis for all patients with diabetes, with a requirement for accurate diabetic patient registers and a target to offer screening to 100% of patients with diabetes by the end of 2007.[22] Digital retinal photography has been chosen as the preferred screening method, largely because it provides excellent retinal images with a high sensitivity and specificity (both >90%), as well as a hard copy of the screen which can be checked and quality assured (QA). The schemes will have standard digital retinal photographs of a macula-, and/or an optic disc-centred view. The English national programme is currently rolling out with 105 schemes involved. At the time of going to press, more schemes will have completed rollout (Figure 3).[21]

Figure 3: The rollout of the English Diabetic Retinopathy Screening Programme with progress shown at four time points.[21]

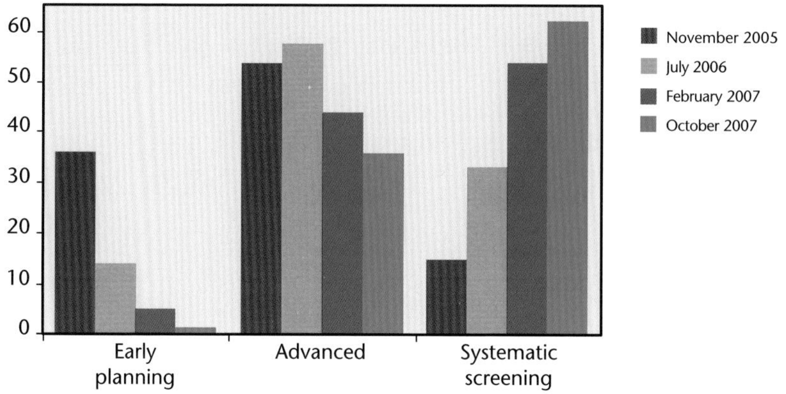

November 2005
July 2006
February 2007
October 2007

Early planning   Advanced   Systematic screening

Adapted with kind permission from the National Screening Committee.

Grading and referrals

Grading of retinal images must be carried out according to three levels of expertise.[23]
- Primary grading: involves the grading of retinal images identifying whether the images are normal or abnormal
- Secondary grading: first full disease grading categorises the precise DR disease level, and second full disease grading, the QA check of all abnormals and 10% of normals
- Tertiary grading: confirms or refines the exact diagnosis, leading to an appropriate clinical action.

A national grading system has been formulated to ensure appropriate referral to diabetic eye services.[21] The grading categories and clinical outcomes will be familiar, but have been allocated a number coding, for example, R1 = background DR.

Maculopathy requiring referral to the diabetic eye service has been defined according to the best surrogate predictors of macular oedema (based on the presence of exudates). Whilst this grading system and categorisation is the one chosen for England, there are variations between the four UK schemes. For example, it is recommended that the common combination of micro-aneurysms within the macular region and normal vision, has annual follow-up in the English scheme, but in other schemes of the four nations, the recommendation is for a 6-monthly retinal re-screen. However, recent data have suggested that only annual follow-up may be required.

Major issues are becoming apparent as the DR digital camera screening programme is evolving, including;

- Queries concerning the accuracy of diabetic patient registers
- Questions such as:
  - Should all patients with diabetes be screened on an annual basis and through dilated pupils?
  - What is the exact prevalence of DR?
  - Are there ethnic differences in prevalence?
  - Can eye departments cope with the number of screen-positive patients, which may be as much as 10% of those initially screened?
  - How much and to what degree of QA is needed for the national scheme?
  - What, if any, is the significance of 1 or 2 micro-aneurysms?
  - Should screening be performed annually or every 2 years for patients with no retinopathy?

Annual screening for DR is the preferred option for patients in view of the logistics and current screening software programming. Initial data from screening programmes and the United Kingdom Asian Diabetes Study (UKADS) show that the prevalence of any DR is 40% in a diabetic population,[24] and that there are ethnic differences (Table 2).

Table 2: Prevalence rates of DR and referral rates for a well established, digital camera-screened diabetic population, a newly digital-screened population in South Birmingham, and from the UKADS in Birmingham and Coventry.[24]

	Established*	New digital[18]	Asian[24]
Normal (R0)	57%	47%	54.4%
Maculopathy (M1)	4.9%	7.5%	12.7%
Pre-proliferative (R2)	3%	1.1%	1%
Proliferative (R3)	1%	1.2%	3%
Referral rate	4%	10%	16.4%
Ungradable	1.8%	2%	–

*Author, personal communication

It is apparent that the onset of accurate digital camera screening is associated with a high rate of referrals to diabetic eye services. In the Asian population in the UK, the prevalence of referable maculopathy may be almost double that of a comparable white Caucasian population.[24] To put this into context, in the Birmingham and Black Country Diabetic Retinopathy Screening Programme[25] there are 90,000 patients with diabetes currently on the database, with the expectation of approximately 7,500 patients being referred into diabetic eye departments in the first year, which will be greater in areas with high Asian diabetic prevalence. For eye departments to cope with this initial workload will pose a major challenge, but this can be alleviated by the use of early re-photographic surveillance and follow-up. Our experience has suggested that this will absorb approximately 25% of eye clinic referrals (author, personal communication).

Quality assurance

QA, regular reports and audits will underpin the whole national DR screening programme, with checks required at each stage of the screening process.[21] It is noteworthy that a number of the QA targets relate not only to the screening process but to the timings and outcomes of diabetic eye services. In addition, there are requirements for appropriate timing of laser therapy as well as recording of visual outcomes. To achieve the QA targets will require close liaison between diabetes and eye departments, so that the national DR screening programme can move towards a diabetic eye disease management programme, which is the long-term aim to improve patient care and outcomes.[21] This is therefore a hot topic for clinicians, primary care trusts and hospital management to ensure appropriate data collection, services and funding are in place.

The National Screening Committee (NSC) has outlined the QA standard of re-grading 10% of all normal and abnormal images at first full-disease grading level.[21] This view has been challenged with QA over a 2-year period, re-grading a random sample of 12% of images of people reported to have retinopathy and of 2% reported as normal, which the authors concluded was a robust and cost-effective system, with particular emphasis on the cost.[26] However, this statement was challenged by the QA lead for the English National Programme, who stated that effective performance monitoring requires a table of basic statistics, including total patients diagnosed, and numbers of eligible, invited, attending, graded, referred and treated patients.[27] Only then is it appropriate to assess quality of grading, as a whole, and by an individual screener.[27] The latter was stressed since the national system of QA is essential to compare different programmes against the same standards, rather than allowing them to present only the data that shows them in the best possible light.

The initial finding arising from schemes using the NSC QA requirements is that although they appear costly, there has been a definite advantage, with clinical misses of sight threatening DR being picked up by QA grading, which is particularly important in the early stages of screening schemes when skills of the first full disease graders are being monitored and improved.[28] The QA system allows for an assessment of each grader's skills at an early stage, allowing feedback and improved performance. In the first weeks of our scheme, QA and arbitration grading detected 61 clinical misses of predominantly diabetic maculopathy, such that feedback and in some cases further training of screeners has quickly ensured a safe and effective screening process (author, personal communication). There are also cost savings related to the accuracy of grading assured by QA, as it ensures that only the correct and appropriate referrals are made to diabetic eye specialists.

The debate continues over the significance of one or two identified micro-aneurysms, thereby constituting background retinopathy. A recent report from the US Diabetes Prevention Program has shown that DR is detected in 7.9% of subjects with impaired glucose tolerance, thus implying that retinal lesions characteristic of diabetes are present in people with elevated fasting glucose and impaired glucose tolerance and no known history of diabetes, and increase in prevalence very early in the course of diabetes.[29] The authors also suggest that the current criteria for diagnosis of diabetes may require further consideration, and that earlier screening for retinopathy in the pre-diabetic state is warranted.[29] These suggestions would have profound implications for both diabetes care and DR screening programmes.

This, however, is challenged by observations of the prevalence of retinopathy in non-diabetic populations. In a recent report of the Blue Mountains Eye Study of 3,654 residents aged over 49 years of age, there was a 5-year cumulative incidence of 9.5% of any retinopathy, with a rate of 7.2% for the development of one or more micro-aneurysms in the retina.[30] This population did not have glucose tolerance testing, but did exclude patients who were known to have diabetes and those with established retinovascular disease (e.g., retinal vein occlusion) from the analysis. This study has recorded a rate of micro-aneurysm detection close to that obtained in the Diabetes Prevention Programme[31] and suggests that one or two micro-aneurysms may not signify DR.[30] Interestingly, the Blue Mountain study showed that 72.3% of retinopathic changes resolved over the 5-year period of observation.[30]

Conclusion

DR is still one of the most common causes of blindness worldwide, despite available proven medical and ophthalmologic treatments. Research continues to demonstrate exciting new therapeutic options, such as lipid lowering, PKC inhibition, and intravitreal anti-VEGF treatments.

All healthcare professionals involved in diabetes care will become involved to some extent in the new National DR Screening Programme. Correct implementation will undoubtedly save vision in people with diabetes, should have a major impact on the reduction in blindness within our diabetic population, and should be cost effective. It will be the duty of all healthcare professionals involved in diabetes care, for example, diabetologists, ophthalmologists, general practitioners, optometrists, diabetes specialist nurses, practice nurses, and the empowered patient with diabetes, to be involved in making sure that all people with diabetes have an annual DR digital retinal photographic screen, so that they are seen in diabetic eye clinics at an early stage to allow for the maximum benefit from laser and other treatments.

References

1.   Brownlee M. Biochemistry and molecular cell biology of diabetic complications. *Nature* 2001; **414**: 813–20.

2.   Donaldson M, Dodson PM. Medical treatment of diabetic retinopathy *Eye* 2003; **17**: 550–62.

3.   Frank RN. Diabetic retinopathy. *N Engl J Med* 2004; **350**: 48–58.

4.   Chaturvedi N, Sjolie AK, Stephenson JM *et al*. Effect of lisinopril on progression of retinopathy in normotensive people with type 1 diabetes. The EUCLID Study Group. EURODIAB Controlled Trial of Lisinopril in Insulin-Dependent Diabetes Mellitus. *Lancet* 1998; **351**: 28–31.

5.   Chaturvedi N, Sjoelie AK, Svensson A; DIRECT Programme Study Group. The DIabetic Retinopathy Candesartan Trials (DIRECT) Programme, rationale and study design. *J Renin Angiotensin Aldosterone Syst* 2002; **3**: 255–61.

6.   Koya D, King GL. Protein kinase C activation and the development of diabetic complications. *Diabetes* 1998; **47**: 859–66.

7. The PKC–DRS Study Group. The effect of ruboxistaurin on visual loss in patients with moderately severe to very severe non-proliferative diabetic retinopathy. Initial results of the protein kinase C β inhibitor retinopathy study (PKC–DRS) multicenter randomised clinical trial. *Diabetes* 2005; **54**: 2188–97.

8. The PKC-DMES Study Group; Aiello LP, David MD *et al*. Effect of ruboxistaurin in patients with diabetic macular edema: thirty-month results of the randomized PKC-DMES clinical trial. *Arch Ophthalmol* 2007; **125**: 318–24.

9. The PKC–DRS 2 Study Group. The effect of ruboxistaurin on visual loss in patients with diabetic retinopathy. *Ophthalmology* 2006; **113**: 2221–30.

10. Eli Lilly Press Release. 18th August 2006. http://www.prnewswire.com/cgi-bin/ micro_stories.pl?ACCT=916306&TICK=LLY&STORY=/www/story/08-18-2006/0004418435&EDATE=Aug+18,+2006 (Last accessed 17.09.07).

11. Chowdhury TA, Hopkins D, Dodson PM, Vafidis GC. The role of serum lipids in exudative diabetic maculopathy: is there a place for lipid lowering? *Eye* 2002; **16**: 689–93.

12. Duncan LJ, Cullen JF, Ireland JT *et al*. A three-year trial of atromid therapy in exudative diabetic retinopathy. *Diabetes* 1968; **17**: 458–67.

13. Cullen JF, Ireland JT, Oliver MF. A controlled trial of Atromid therapy in exudative diabetic retinopathy. *Trans Ophthalmol Soc UK* 1964; **84**: 281–95.

14. Chew EY, Klein ML, Ferris FL *et al*. Association of elevated serum lipid levels with retinal hard exudate in diabetic retinopathy. Early Treatment Diabetic Retinopathy Study (ETDRS) Report 22. *Arch Ophthalmol* 1996; **114**: 1079–84.

15. Miljanovic B, Glynn RJ, Nathan DM *et al*. A prospective study of serum lipids and risk of diabetic macular oedema in type 1 diabetes *Diabetes* 2004; **53**: 2883–92.

16. Song W, Barth JL, Lu K *et al*. Effects of modified low-density lipoproteins on human retinal pericyte survival. *Ann N Y Acad Sci* 2005; **1043**: 390–5.

17. Kim J, Ahn JH, Kim JH *et al*. Fenofibrate regulates retinal endothelial cell survival through the AMPK signal transduction pathway. *Exp Eye Res* 2007; **84**: 886–93.

18. Colhoun HM, Betteridge DJ, Durington PN *et al*. Primary prevention of cardiovascular disease with atorvastatin in type 2 diabetes in the Collaborative Atorvastatin Diabetes Study (CARDS): multicentre randomised placebo-controlled trial. *Lancet* 2004; **364**: 685–96.

19. Chew EY, Ambrosius WT, Howard LT *et al*. Rationale, design,and methods of the action to control cardiovascular risk in Diabetes eye study (ACCORD–EYE). *Am J Cardiol* 2007; **99**: 103i–111i.

20. The FIELD Study Investigators. Effects of long-term fenofibrate on cardiovascular events in 9,795 people with type 2 diabetes mellitus (the FIELD study): randomised controlled trial. *Lancet* 2005; **366**: 1849–61.

21. A National Screening Programme for Sight Threatening Diabetic Retinopathy. http://www.nscretinopathy.org.uk/ (Last accessed 18.09.07).

22. Diabetes UK. http://www.diabetes.org.uk/About_us/Our_Views/Position_statements/Retinal_screening/ (Last accessed 18.09.07).

23. Scottish Diabetes Retinopathy Screening Service. http://www.scotland.gov.uk/Publications/2003/07/17638/23077 (Last accessed 18.09.07).

24. PKC-DRS2 Group. Effect of ruboxistaurin on visual loss in patients with diabetic retinopathy. *Ophthalmology* 2006; **113**: 2221–30.

25. The Birmingham and Black Country Diabetic Retinopathy Screening Programme. http://wwwretinopathyscreening.co.uk (Last accessed 18.09.07).

26. Arun CS, Young D, Batey D *et al*. Establishing ongoing quality assurance in a retinal screening programme *Diabetic Med* 2006; **23**: 629–34.

27. Garvican L. Issues regarding quality assurance in the English National Screening Programme for sight threatening diabetic retinopathy; response to paper by Arun C *et al*. *Diabetic Medicine* 2007; **24**: 688–9.

28. Whitehouse KH, Seymour HC, Leigh R *et al*. How important is arbitration grading upon both grading and feral within a digital diabetic retinopathy screening programme. Presented at ABCD meeting, Chester, UK May 2007.

29. Diabetes Prevention Program Research Group. The prevalence of retinopathy in impaired glucose tolerance and recent onset diabetes in the Diabetes Prevention Program. *Diabetic Med* 2007; **24**: 137–44.

30. Cugati S, Cikamatana L, Wang JJ *et al*. Five-year incidence and progression of vascular retinopathy in persons without diabetes; the Blue Mountains Eye Study. *Eye* 2006; **20**: 1239–45.

31. Diabetes Prevention Program Research Group. Reduction in the incidence of type 2 diabetes with lifestyle intervention or metformin. *N Engl J Med* 2002; **346**: 393–403.

New drug therapies for diabetic retinopathy

Professor Simon Harding

Key points

- Optical coherence tomography is an important new tool for assessing the indications for new treatments for diabetic maculopathy and monitoring their effectiveness.
- Monoclonal antibodies against vascular endothelial growth factor (VEGF) show great promise in the management of diabetic retinopathy, but conclusive clinical trial evidence is awaited.
- The use of pegaptanib sodium and ranibizumab is unlikely to be approved by funding agencies for clinical practice outside trials.
- Bevacizumab, a less expensive anti-VEGF drug, may prove useful as an adjunct to established treatments for severe and refractory cases.
- The mainstay of management of diabetic retinopathy and maculopathy remains argon laser photocoagulation.

Introduction

Diabetic retinopathy affects vision through the development of retinal neovascularisation and maculopathy. Maculopathy occurs in three forms: focal exudative, diffuse and ischaemic. Typically each eye exhibits more than one form. Current management relies on argon laser photocoagulation, which is highly effective in the prevention of visual loss from proliferative retinopathy, but not as effective in maculopathy, especially in cases in which diffuse and ischaemic features predominate. There is therefore a need to develop new drugs to prevent visual loss in patients with maculopathy.

Key pathological processes in the development of diabetic retinopathy and maculopathy are centred on the retinal capillary with the development of non-perfusion and leakage. Non-perfusion leads to tissue hypoxia with a subsequent drive to angiogenesis. Leakage is caused by increased vascular permeability and inflammation; the latter is also implicated in capillary non-perfusion through increased leukocyte adhesion. The proteins and growth factors involved in these processes, including vascular endothelial growth factor (VEGF) and inflammatory cytokines, are targets for drug therapy.

The morphological features of diabetic macular oedema can be observed using optical coherence tomography (OCT), which is now widely used in the management and follow-up of patients, especially if refractory to laser therapy. Typical features visible on OCT are thickening of the retina and the presence of intraretinal cysts, as shown in Figure 1.

Figure 1: Optical coherence tomography report including images of an eye with cystoid macular oedema showing increased central retinal thickness, the presence of intra-retinal cysts and an attached posterior vitreous face.

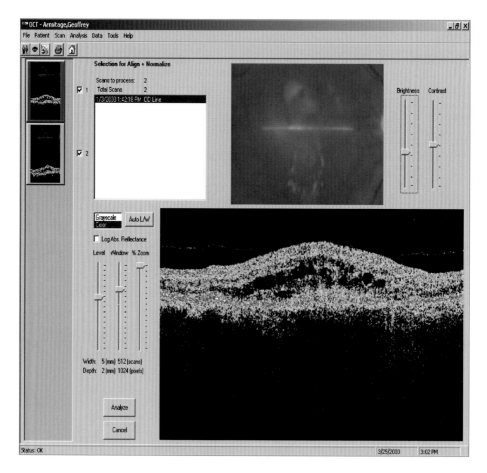

The thickness of the retina is usually measured as an average of the central segment on a thickness map and is termed the central retinal thickness (CRT). Attachment of the posterior face of the vitreous can also be seen, and, if present, vitreous surgery can be considered.

Anti-VEGF therapy

VEGF has been identified as a key protein involved in the pathological processes of diabetic retinopathy through its actions in increasing vascular permeability, angiogenesis, and inflammation.[1] Several anti-VEGF drugs are currently under investigation, mainly for the treatment of choroidal neovascularisation in age-related macular degeneration (AMD), with three being introduced into clinical practice: pegaptanib sodium, ranibizumab and bevacizumab. These drugs are also being trialled in patients with diabetic retinopathy. The route of administration used is injection into the vitreous cavity of the eye.

Pegaptanib sodium is a pegylated aptamer that binds to VEGF receptors, with specific selectivity for the 165 isoform. Pegaptanib sodium has been investigated in diabetic maculopathy by the Macugen Diabetic Retinopathy Study Group.[2] In this phase II, randomised, clinical trial, 172 patients were randomly allocated to four groups to receive three, 6-weekly injections of active drug at doses of 0.3, 1.0 or 3.0 mg, or sham injections. Results reported an improvement in median visual acuity (VA) at week 36 with the 0.3 mg dose [best-corrected VA (BCVA): 20/50] compared with sham (20/63) (p = 0.04). Significantly more patients in the 0.3 mg group experienced an improvement in vision [≥10 letters on an Early Treatment Diabetic Retinopathy Study (ETDRS) chart] at 36 weeks compared with sham (34% vs. 10%, p = 0.003), and there were trend improvements in frequency of visual improvement and reduced CRT on OCT. The effect on proliferative retinopathy was investigated in a small subgroup analysis from this study and retinal neovascularisation was observed in 19 of the 172 patients.[3] Regression occurred in 8 of 13 (62%) in the pegaptanib-treated group and 0 of 3 in the sham group.

Ranibizumab is a humanised monoclonal antibody that targets all isoforms of VEGF. The drug has been studied in a small pilot study in ten eyes of ten patients with centre-threatening maculopathy.[4] During the trial, patients received three, 4-weekly injections of the drug. Vision improvement (≥15 letters) was observed at 3 months in four patients and there was a mean decrease in CRT of 197.8 ± 85 μm in all five patients in the 0.5 mg dose group.

Bevacizumab, the parent molecule from which ranibizumab is derived, is licensed for use in the treatment of colonic carcinoma. As a result of its size (full-length antibody), it has a longer half-life in the eye than ranibizumab (20 days vs. 4 hours). Being a larger molecule it may not penetrate the retina to the same extent as ranibizumab, although one study in 6 cynomolgous monkeys demonstrated its presence in inner retina and choroid as quickly as 1 day after intraocular injection.[5] Bevacizumab binds to all biologically-active VEGF isoforms.[6] Since the Fc portion of immunoglobulin IgG is retained in bevacizumab, it poses a potentially higher risk of post-injection intraocular inflammation, compared with ranibizumab. The main attraction of the drug is that the cost is considerably less than ranibizumab.

To date, the only published data on the use of bevacizumab in diabetic maculopathy have been from case series. Arevalo and colleagues reported a multicentre, retrospective case series of 110 eyes of 88 consecutive patients with diabetic macular oedema receiving 1.25 mg or 2.5 mg of bevacizumab, followed for a mean 6.31 ± 0.8 months.[7] Following treatment, there were significant improvements in BCVA, measured using a logMAR chart (baseline 0.87, final 0.6, p<0.0001) and CRT on OCT testing (baseline 387.0 ± 182.8 μm, final 275.7 ± 108.3 μm, p<0.0001). Haritoglou and co-workers reported a prospective case series of 51 patients with centre-involved diffuse diabetic macular oedema treated with 1.25 mg bevacizumab.[8] Of the 23 patients to complete 12 weeks of follow-up, 16 (70%) received two or more injections. At 12 weeks, there was a significant reduction in CRT compared with placebo, but no detectable change in mean VA (p = 0.001).

Two small case series' have been reported to date investigating the use of bevacizumab in patients with proliferative diabetic retinopathy (PDR) and advanced disease. In the first, reduced leakage on fluorescein angiography was seen in 15 patients with PDR refractory to laser photocoagulation, treated with a single dose of 1.5 mg bevacizumab.[9] Avery and colleagues reported partial or complete resolution of retinal, disc or iris neovascularisation in 44 eyes of 44 patients treated with a range of doses between 0.625 and 1.25 mg, with a response seen at week 1.[10] There is also evidence to support the future use of bevacizumab in the management of neovascular glaucoma;[11] however, further studies are needed.

There are a number of limitations with the emerging anti-VEGF drugs in the treatment of diabetic retinopathy. In the absence of randomised, clinical trial data, their use must be considered experimental, although some of the early experience is encouraging. Clinicians need to understand that the drug is unlicensed for use in the eye and any administration is "off-label".

Effects on vision appear to be less dramatic than those of the morphological appearance on OCT. The frequency and duration of treatment remains uncertain. Experience from the PIER study of ranibizumab in AMD (unpublished data) shows that any initial benefit on VA and OCT appearance is likely to wear off after approximately 6 months. In addition, there are important cost considerations associated with the use of pegaptanib and ranibizumab.

Safety concerns with the use of anti-VEGF agents are currently not an issue, but solid data from large trials is lacking. In treatment trials in AMD, there has been a small increase in the incidence of stroke and therefore caution should be exercised in the frequent use of anti-VEGF agents in patients with cardiovascular disease. Caution should also be exercised in women of child-bearing age as there have also been a small number of reports of amenorrhea (which is of greater importance in patients with diabetes than AMD). In the case series reported by Avery and co-workers[10] there was an observed effect on macular oedema in the fellow eyes of patients with bilateral disease, indicating a definite systemic action.

The most significant risk with the use of bevacizumab is of endophthalmitis, a potentially devastating intraocular infection in the vitreous. In the Macugen Diabetic Retinopathy Study, 0.8% of patients developed endophthalmitis.[2] Great care is required to prevent endophthalmitis, and is achieved through the use of an aseptic technique, careful draping, the use of a speculum and antibiotic drops post-injection. There is also an additional risk of cataract formation. In the longer term, there are concerns regarding the effect of bevacizumab on capillary non-perfusion and the impact on VEGF receptors on neurons and astrocytes in the eye. Powerful VEGF blockade may increase apoptosis of photoreceptors and ganglion cells. It is possible that an advantage of selective blockade with pegaptanib over total blockade with ranibizumab and bevacizumab, may be shown in the future.

Developments with other drugs

Intravitreal triamcinolone acetate (IVTA) steroid injection is still used fairly widely by ophthalmologists in clinical practice. However, to date, there has been no convincing evidence of effectiveness on VA in any ocular disease. Most reports have been short case series and have reported improvements in OCT appearance but not vision. In addition, serious concern has been raised regarding the development of glaucoma, which has been observed in up to 40% of patients, and of the induction of cataract, as demonstrated in the study by Islam and colleagues.[12]

One recent, medium-sized randomised, controlled trial compared intravitreal injections of 4 mg of triamcinolone acetate with further argon laser photocoagulation in 88 eyes with persistent, clinically significant macular oedema, who had received at least one previous episode of laser.[13] Improvement of 15 or more ETDRS letters was seen in 2 of 41 patients in the IVTA group (4.9%) and in 5 out of 41 (12.2%) patients in the laser group; the difference did not reach statistical significance (p = 0.49). There were no other statistically significant differences between the groups detected in the study outcomes – mean VA score or CRT on OCT. There was one case of sterile endophthalmitis and 22 out of 43 patients in the IVTA group required treatment for glaucoma.

Ruboxistaurin, which blocks the β isoform of protein kinase C, remains a drug with considerable potential, but to date has not been licensed for use in the treatment of patients with diabetic retinopathy. The most promising results to date have come from the MBCM trial in which 685 patients with moderate-to-severe pre-proliferative diabetic retinopathy were randomised to receive either 32 mg of ruboxistaurin (n = 345) or placebo (n = 340).[14] There was a 40% risk reduction in sustained moderate visual loss ($\geq$15 ETDRS letters on more than one occasion, p = 0.034): 5.5% in the treated group and 9.1% in the placebo group. Ruboxistaurin-treated patients experienced significantly better mean VA and frequency of visual improvement compared with placebo (p = 0.005). There was also significantly less progression to clinically significant macular oedema and to first laser treatment (p = 0.003). The application for a licence has been rejected by the US Food and Drug Administration who have requested further clinical trial evidence.

Somatostatin (octeotride) has been studied in two large, randomised, clinical trials the results of which are yet to be published. Negative results caused the discontinuation of the drug-development programme.

Conclusions

Drug therapies for diabetic retinopathy offer considerable promise for the future. The role of anti-VEGF therapies needs to be developed further and there is an urgent need for randomised clinical trials. It appears that their main role at this stage will be in the treatment of persistent and refractory macular oedema and proliferative diabetic retinopathy. Triamcinolone is still being used widely, mainly because of reduced costs, but the potential for side effects will likely limit its use once improved therapies are developed. However, in this time of considerable interest in pharmacological agents, it is important to recognise that the mainstay of therapy for diabetic retinopathy remains argon laser photocoagulation, which if applied competently, still offers proven benefit for the majority of patients.

References

1. Aiello LP. Vascular endothelial growth factor. 20th Century mechanisms, 21st Century therapies. *Invest Ophthalmol Vis Sci* 1997; **38**: 1647–52.

2. Cunningham ET, Adamis AP, Altaweel M *et al.* and the Macugen Diabetic Retinopathy Study Group. A phase II randomised double-masked trial of pegaptanib, an anti-vascular endothelial growth factor aptamer, for diabetic macular edema. *Ophthalmology* 2005; **112**: 23–28.

3. Adamis AP, Altaweel M, Bressler NM *et al.* and the Macugen Diabetic Retinopathy Study Group. Changes in retinal neovascularization after pegaptanib (Macugen) therapy in diabetic individuals. *Ophthalmology* 2007; **114**: 615–6.

4. Chun DW, Heier JS, Topping TM *et al.* A pilot study of multiple intravitreal injections of ranibizumab in patients with center-involving clinically significant diabetic macular edema. *Ophthalmology* 2006; **113**: 1706–12.

5. Heiduschka P, Fietz H, Hofmeister S *et al.* and the Tübingen Bevacizumab Study Group. Penetration of bevacizumab through the retina after intravitreal injection in the monkey. *Invest Ophthalmol Vis Sci* 2007; **48**: 2814–23.

6. Zondor SD, Medina PJ. Bevacizumab: an angiogenesis inhibitor with efficacy in colorectal and other malignancies. *Ann Pharmacother* 2004; **38**: 1258–64.

7. Arevalo JF, Fromow-Guerra J, Quiroz-Mercado H *et al;* Pan-American Collaborative Retina Study Group. Primary intravitreal bevacizumab (Avastin) for diabetic macular edema: results from the Pan-American Collaborative Retina Study Group at 6-month follow-up. *Ophthalmology* 2007; **114**: 743–50.

8. Haritoglou C, Kook D, Neubauer A *et al.* Intravitreal bevacizumab (Avastin) therapy for persistent diffuse diabetic macular edema. *Retina* 2006; **26**: 999–1005.

9. Jorge R, Costa RA, Calucci D *et al.* Intravitreal bevacizumab (Avastin) for persistent new vessels in diabetic retinopathy (IBEPE study). *Retina* 2006; **26**: 1006–13.

10. Avery RL, Pearlman J, Pieramici DJ *et al.* Intravitreal bevacizumab (Avastin) in the treatment of proliferative diabetic retinopathy. *Ophthalmology* 2006; **113**: 1695–1705.

11. Iliev ME, Domig D, Wolf-Schnurrbursch U *et al.* Intravitreal bevacizumab (Avastin) in the treatment of neovascular glaucoma. *Am J Ophthalmol* 2006; **6**: 1054–6.

12. Islam MS, Vernon SA, Negi A. Intravitreal triamcinolone will cause posterior subcapsular cataract in most eyes with diabetic maculopathy within 2 years. *Eye* 2007; **21**: 321–3.

13. Ockrim Z, Sivaprasad S, Falk S *et al.* Intravitreal triamcinolone versus laser photocoagulation for diabetic macular oedema. *Eur J Ophthalmol* 2007; **17**: 474.

14. PKC-DRS2 Group, Aiello LP, Davis MD *et al.* Effect of ruboxistaurin on visual loss in patients with diabetic retinopathy. *Ophthalmology* 2006; **113**: 2221–30.

Advances in the management of painful diabetic neuropathy

Professor Solomon Tesfaye

Key points

- Diabetic peripheral neuropathic pain (DPNP) is under-diagnosed and under-treated. It has a prevalence rate of 16–26% in patients with diabetes.
- The minimum requirements for diagnosis of DPNP are assessment of symptoms and neurological examination, with shoes and socks removed. Bilateral sensory impairment is almost always present.
- DPNP is characterised by burning, shooting or stabbing pain in the extremities. Pain may be spontaneous or evoked.
- Optimisation of cardiovascular risk factors and improved glycaemic control are important.
- First-line therapies for DPNP are a tricyclic antidepressant, serotonin–noradrenaline re-uptake inhibitor (such as duloxetine) or anticonvulsants (such as pregabalin or gabapentin), taking into account patient co-morbidities and cost.
- Combination therapy may be useful, but further research is required.

Introduction

Polyneuropathy is one of the most common complications of diabetes and the most common form of neuropathy in the developed world. Diabetic polyneuropathy encompasses several neuropathic syndromes, the most common of which is chronic distal symmetrical neuropathy, also known as diabetic peripheral neuropathy (DPN), the main initiating factor for foot ulceration.

Diabetic peripheral neuropathy

Epidemiology
Several clinic- and population-based studies show prevalence rates for DPN – approximately 30% of all patients with diabetes – though after 25 years of diabetes, the number of affected patients increases to 50%.[1] The European Diabetes (EURODIAB) Complications Study found a prevalence rate of 28% for distal symmetrical neuropathy in type 1 diabetes.[2] After excluding those with neuropathy at baseline, the study showed that, over a 7-year period, approximately 25% of patients with type 1 diabetes developed DPN, with age, duration of diabetes and poor glycaemic control being the

major disease determinants.[3] Neuropathy was also associated with potentially modifiable cardiovascular risk factors such as serum lipids, blood pressure, body mass index and albumin excretion rate.[3] Based on recent epidemiological studies, correlates of DPN include increasing age, increasing duration of diabetes, poor glycaemic control and cardiovascular risk factors, including hypertension, retinopathy and albuminuria.[1–3]

Diabetic peripheral neuropathic pain

The main clinical presentation of DPN is sensory loss, which the patient may not be aware of, or may describe as 'numbness' or 'dead feeling'. However, some patients may experience a progressive build-up of unpleasant sensory symptoms including: tingling (paraesthesia); burning pain; shooting pains (like 'electric shock') down the legs; lancinating (also likened to 'stabbing' or 'knife-like' pains); contact pain, often with day-time clothes and bedclothes (allodynia); pain on walking, often described as 'walking barefoot on marbles' or 'walking barefoot on hot sand'; sensations of heat or cold in the feet; persistent aching feeling in the feet and cramp-like sensations in the legs. Occasionally, pain can extend above the feet and may involve the whole of the legs. When this occurs, there is usually also upper-limb involvement. There is a large spectrum of severity of these symptoms, with some patients having only minor complaints, such as tingling in one or two toes, whilst others may be affected with devastating complications such as 'the numb diabetic foot' or severe painful neuropathy that does not respond to drug therapy.

Diabetic peripheral neuropathic pain (DPNP) is a common and challenging condition. It is characteristically more severe at night and often prevents sleep.[4] Some patients may be in a constant state of tiredness because of sleep deprivation,[4] whilst others may be unable to maintain full employment. Severe painful neuropathy can occasionally cause marked reduction in exercise threshold, so as to interfere with daily activities. It is therefore not surprising that depressive symptoms are not uncommon.[4]

Epidemiology of DPNP
Despite pain being the most distressing symptom of DPN and the main reason for seeking medical attention, there are few studies specifically examining the prevalence of DPNP. Among these studies, prevalence rates of between 7%–20% have been reported, reflecting differing criteria used to define neuropathic pain.[5] In the EURODIAB prospective study, almost a quarter of patients with neuropathy developed neuropathic symptoms over a 7-year period,[3] indicating that a significant number of patients with diabetes suffer from neuropathic pain.[5]

Acute painful neuropathies
DPNP may present acutely within the context of poor glycaemic control, typically in patients with type 1 diabetes (acute painful neuropathy of poor glycaemic control) or after initiation of treatment (acute painful neuropathy of rapid glycaemic control).[6]

These acute syndromes are relatively rare compared with the chronic painful neuropathy associated with DPN. Within weeks, patients experience a rapid build-up of uncomfortable sensory symptoms, leading to persistent lower-limb burning pain, paraesthesia and allodynia, with nocturnal exacerbation and depression.[6] There may also be marked, precipitous weight loss. Sensory loss is often mild or absent, and there are no motor signs. Complete resolution of symptoms occurs within a year.[6]

Mechanisms of neuropathic pain

Psychological and cultural factors play an important role in the perception and expression of pain. Unlike nociceptive pain, neuropathic pain is caused by dysfunction of the peripheral or central nervous system (CNS) and does not require any receptor stimulation. Painful symptoms are relayed by small myelinated A-δ and unmyelinated C fibres. Unmyelinated C fibres are thought to transmit the slower component of pain, whereas myelinated A-δ fibres relay the faster component.

The exact pathophysiological mechanisms of neuropathic pain in diabetes remain unknown, although several mechanisms, including peripheral and central, correlate with the postulation of painful neuropathy (Table 1).[7]

Table 1: Mechanisms of neuropathic pain.[7]

Peripheral mechanisms	Central mechanisms
Changes in sodium-channel distribution and expression	Central sensitisation
Altered neuro-peptide expression	Aβ fibre sprouting into lamina II of the dorsal horn
Sympathetic sprouting	Reduced inhibition of descending pathways
Peripheral sensitisation	
Altered peripheral blood flow	
Axonal atrophy, degeneration or regeneration	
Damage to small fibres	
Glycaemic flux	

More recently, *in vivo* studies have shown an increase in sural nerve epineurial blood flow in subjects with DPNP compared with those with painless DPN,[8] suggesting that haemodynamic factors may have an important role in the pathogenesis of neuropathic pain and might offer further insight into potential treatments for this distressing condition. Another recent study examined lower-extremity skin intra-epidermal nerve fibres (IENFs) demonstrating severe loss of IENF is associated with the presence of neuropathic pain in patients with little or no objective sign of neuropathy.[9]

A number of peripheral and central mechanisms may explain neuropathic pain (Table 1). It is apparent that the insult of diabetes occurs at all levels of the nervous system, from the peripheral nerve to the brain. There is now also magnetic resonance imaging (MRI) evidence for the involvement of the spinal cord in DPN,[10] apparently at the early (sub-clinical) stage.[11] Lesions in the spinal cord may result in pain syndromes similar to those seen after spinal cord injury or demyelination.[12] In some patients with painful neuropathy, there may be little in the way of abnormalities on clinical examination or electrophysiological parameters, but there may be evidence of marked abnormalities in somatosensory-evoked potentials within the spinal cord.[13] Recently, a study using MR spectroscopy has also demonstrated the presence of thalamic neuronal dysfunction in painless but not painful DPN, suggesting that a functioning thalamus – the gateway to all sensory information – is required in order to perceive pain.[14] It is thus increasingly clear that the impact of diabetes on the nervous system is far more generalised than previously thought. Modern imaging techniques are currently investigating the full extent of involvement of the CNS in both DPN and DPNP.

Recent advances in the management of DPNP

The pharmacological management of DPNP has recently been reviewed by a consensus panel.[5] The assessment and management of neuropathic pain continues to pose a considerable challenge to clinicians.[4,5,7] A careful history and peripheral neurologi-cal/vascular examination of the patient is essential in order to exclude other possible causes of leg pain, such as peripheral vascular disease, prolapsed intervertebral discs, spinal-canal stenosis and *corda equina* lesions. Unilateral leg pain should arouse suspi-cion that the pain may be due to lumbar–sacral nerve-root compression. These patients may well need to undergo investigation with lumbar–sacral MRI. Quality and severity should be assessed, preferably using a suitable pain rating scale, so that response to treatment may be evaluated. Most importantly, an empathic approach with multidisciplinary support is crucial as the psychological impact of DPNP is considerable.[4]

There is now little doubt that improved glycaemic control is central to prevent-ing/delaying the onset of DPN. However, there are no controlled studies that show the efficacy of good glycaemic control in reducing pain perception. Nevertheless, despite the lack of well-designed studies in this area, there is a general consensus that intensive blood glucose control should be the first step in the treatment of any form of diabetic polyneuropathy. Traditional markers of large vessel disease, including hypertension, obesity, hyperlipidaemia and smoking, also appear to be independent risk factors for DPN[3] and therefore also need to be effectively managed by life-style change and pharmacotherapy.

Pharmacological treatment

Pharmacological treatment of DPNP is not entirely satisfactory as currently available drugs may not be effective and may be complicated by side effects.[5] The range of therapies currently under investigation include: tricyclic compounds (e.g. amitriptyline 25–150 mg/day; imipramine 25–100 mg/day), selective serotonin–noradrenaline-reuptake inhibitors (SNRIs e.g. duloxetine 60–120 mg/day; venlafaxine 150–225 mg/day), anticonvulsants (e.g. carbamazepine 200–800 mg/day; gabapentin 300–3600 mg/day; pregabalin 300–600 mg/day); opiates (tramadol 200–400 mg/day; morphine sulphate SR 20–80 mg/day; oxycodone 20–80 mg/day), membrane stabilisers including mexiletine and intravenous lignocaine; the antioxidant, α-lipoic acid and the substance-P depleter, topical capsaicin. However, despite these therapies, the treatment scenario remains less than satisfactory, with many sufferers having sub-optimal pain relief.[5] Moreover, only two agents (duloxetine and pregabalin) are formally approved by the US Food and Drug Administration for the treatment of DPNP.

Tricyclic antidepressants

Tricyclic antidepressants (TCAs) block reuptake of serotonin (5-hydroxytryptamine, 5-HT) and noradrenaline, and also block sodium and calcium channels. In a placebo-controlled, 6-week cross-over study, 74% of patients with DPNP obtained at least 50% pain relief with amitriptyline compared with 41% for placebo.[15] However, the TCAs also have many side effects particularly anti-cholinergic effects such as dry mouth, sedation, sweating and dizziness. Treatment is ideally started at night, when neuropathic pain is worse, to assist with sleep. This should ideally be started at a small dose of, for example, 25 mg before bed, and gradually titrated depending on side-effects and efficacy. TCAs can cause hypotension that can incapacitate patients with orthostatic hypotension as a result of autonomic neuropathy. Recent data from a retrospective study including 58,956 person-years of follow-up on TCA therapy indicate an increased risk of sudden cardiac death associated with TCA doses in excess of 100 mg/day.[16] As a result, TCAs may be contra-indicated in some patients with type 2 diabetes with co-morbidities such as cardiovascular disease.

Selective serotonin–noradrenaline-reuptake inhibitors (SNRIs)

SNRIs, including duloxetine and venlafaxine, increase synaptic availability of 5-HT and noradrenaline in the descending pathways that are inhibitory to pain impulses. In patients with diabetes and DPNP, randomised to duloxetine, 20, 60 and 120 mg/day or placebo, treatment with duloxetine 60 mg/day or 120 mg/day for 12 weeks produced a significantly greater improvement in the 24-hour average pain score compared with placebo (p<0.05), starting within a week and continuing throughout the trial.[17] These results have been confirmed in two similar-sized trials.[5] Pooled data from all three trials, including a total of 1,139 patients, showed that 45–55% of patients achieved ≥50% pain reduction over 12 weeks of treatment.[5] The number needed to treat (NNT) to achieve at least 50% pain reduction was 4.9 for 120 mg, and 5.2 for 60 mg of duloxetine.[5] Therapy with duloxetine produces no weight gain during treatment for up to a year.

In a 6-week study comparing placebo, venlafaxine 75 mg/day and 150–225 mg/day in 244 patients with diabetes and DPNP, the extent of pain relief achieved in the higher-dose group was similar to that shown with duloxetine.[18] Side effects included somnolence and nausea. In addition, seven patients treated with venlafaxine developed clinically important electrocardiographic changes,[18] which is a major concern given that many patients with diabetes have coincident cardiac disease. Venlafaxine is currently not licensed for use in DPNP.

Anticonvulsants
Anticonvulsants act either by blocking sodium channels or binding to calcium ion channels. Gabapentin and pregabalin act by binding to the α-2-δ sub-unit of the calcium channel, thus reducing calcium flux and neurotransmitter release in the hyper-excited neurone.

In a study comparing gabapentin, titrated from 900 mg/day to 3,600 mg/day over 4 weeks (followed by maintenance at the maximum dose for an additional 4 weeks), with placebo,[19] 59.5% of patients in the treatment arm, 67% of whom received the highest dose of gabapentin, achieved at least a moderate improvement in pain on the patient global impression of change score, compared with placebo (32.9%) There is stronger evidence for the efficacy of pregabalin in DPNP compared with placebo.[5] A combined analysis of six controlled trials of 5–12 weeks duration demonstrated 39% and 46% of patients with DPNP treated with pregabalin 300 mg/day and 600 mg/day, respectively, achieved at least 50% pain relief. Although there are no head-to-head trials comparing pregabalin and duloxetine, the NNTs for their higher doses (i.e. pregabalin 600 mg/day and duloxetine 120 mg/day) appear similar.[17,20]

Opioid agonists
Opioid agonists modulate pain by acting at the peripheral nociceptor, presynaptic receptor, enkephalin interneurons, post-synaptic receptors and surpaspinally, as well as on the descending systems.

Clinical evidence to support the traditional approach of using opioid agonists as add-on to other therapy is limited. In one cross-over study, with nearly half of 40 patients without prior treatment for painful neuropathy, low-dose combination therapy with gabapentin and morphine was significantly more effective than either monotherapy at a higher dose (p<0.05). However, in clinical practice, patients would usually receive pain treatment before an opioid agonist was added.[21] Combination treatment was associated with a higher frequency of adverse effects than either monotherapy.[22]

Lacosamide
In a phase II study, the anticonvulsant lacosamide was found to be beneficial in relieving pain in DPNP, but phase III studies are now required.[23]

α-lipoic acid

There is some evidence that α-lipoic acid is effective in symptomatic neuropathy. A meta-analysis including 1,258 patients from four prospective trials showed that treatment with α-lipoic acid (600 mg/day) for 3 weeks was associated with significant improvement in neuropathic symptoms, as well as neuropathic deficits (p<0.05).[24] Oral treatment with α-lipoic acid for 5 weeks improved neuropathic symptoms and deficits in patients with DPN.[25] An oral dose of 600 mg once-daily appears to provide the optimum risk-to-benefit ratio.[25]

Comparison of the safety and efficacy of available treatments

One method of comparing safety and efficacy across the range of available treatments is by estimation of the NNT and number needed to harm (NNH).[26] The NNT is defined as the number of patients needed to treat with a certain drug to obtain one patient with 50% pain relief.[26] The NNH is defined as the number of patients that need to be treated for one patient to drop out of a study as a result of adverse effects.[26] Though this is a useful approach it is not ideal as many of the trials have different designs, end points etc.

Figure 1 shows a comparison of the NNTs for the various drugs evaluated in painful neuropathy including DPNP. The size of circles indicates the total number of patients used in the trials.

Figure 1: Comparison of the relative efficacy of treatments for painful neuropathic pain (including DPNP), based on NNT.[5]

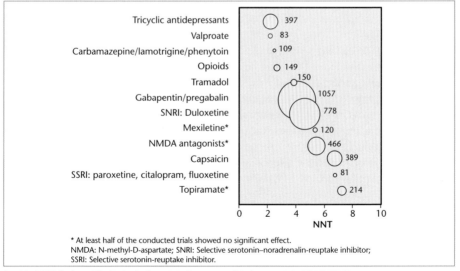

* At least half of the conducted trials showed no significant effect.
NMDA: N-methyl-D-aspartate; SNRI: Selective serotonin–noradrenalin-reuptake inhibitor;
SSRI: Selective serotonin-reuptake inhibitor.

TCAs have the lowest NNTs,[26] although some of the clinical trials were cross-over, thus reducing the NNTs. TCAs also have increased risk of adverse side effects, including dry mouth, sweating, dizziness and sedation, as well as clear contra-indications for use in patients with heart disease, epilepsy and glaucoma.[5,26] Duloxetine, pregabalin and gabapentin have used the largest numbers of patients in trials and appear to have similar intermediate efficacy (Figure 1). Side effects, including dizziness and somnolence, are more common for pregabalin and gabapentin than duloxetine, whereas nausea is more common with duloxetine.[5] In addition, oedema is more common with gabapentin and pregabalin, and duloxetine is contra-indicated in patients with liver disease.[5]

Pharmacological treatment algorithm

The ideal treatment for DPNP results in clinically significant and sustained pain relief, is well tolerated and is inexpensive. Importantly also, treatment should not be associated with negative effects on quality of life, mood, functionality and sleep. The following algorithm was suggested by a panel of experts who carefully evaluated the above attributes for the various drugs.[5]

Comparison of the relative efficacy and safety of treatments for DPNP, based on the available NNT for neuropathic pain (including DPNP) and NNH data, indicates that a TCA, SNRI or an α-2-δ agonist should be considered for first-line treatment of pain in patients with DPNP (Figure 2).

On the basis of trial data, pregabalin would be the preferred α-2-δ-agonist blocker and duloxetine the preferred SNRI. Initially, treatment selection would largely depend on other contra-indications and co-morbidities in the patient, in addition to cost considerations. In patients with diabetes and a history of heart disease, elderly patients on other medications such as diuretics and patients with co-morbid orthostatic hypotension, TCAs are not recommended. The use of pregabalin and gabapentin should be avoided in the presence of oedema, and duloxetine with liver disease. Following the start of treatment, patients should be asked at each visit whether their pain has improved, worsened, or remained unchanged. A simple questionnaire or visual analogue scale may assist in monitoring treatment response. If pain is inadequately controlled, depending on contra-indications, another first-line agent may be considered as shown in Figure 2.

Currently, there is little evidence on which to base decisions for combination therapy. Combination therapy may be considered where pain control is inadequately managed with opioid agonist monotherapy (Figure 2). Caution should be maintained with use of opioids in patients with depression, and these agents should be avoided in patients with a history of substance abuse.

Figure 2: Proposed treatment algorithm for DPNP.[5]

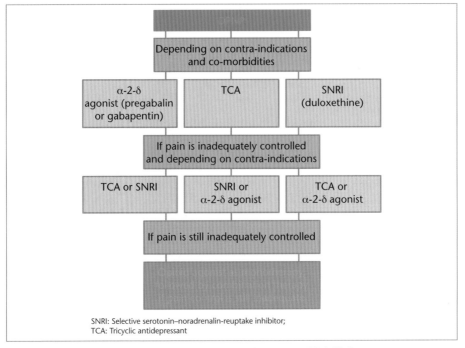

SNRI: Selective serotonin–noradrenalin-reuptake inhibitor;
TCA: Tricyclic antidepressant

Conclusions

DPN and DPNP are important complications of diabetes, with implications for patient morbidity and mortality. Although estimates suggest that DPNP affects approximately 10–20% of diabetic patients, further data from larger, preferably population-based trials, with robust assessments of pain and quality of life, are required. Currently, DPNP is under-diagnosed and under-treated[27] and this has got to change. There is also a need for further research into the mechanisms (e.g. pain processing in the CNS) of DPNP that may result in more effective therapies with fewer side effects.

Recent developments have resulted in the availability of new, effective treatments for DPNP, with improved tolerability compared with the TCAs. However, cost may be an issue. Direct head-to-head comparative trials are required, along with studies into long-term efficacy of drugs. There is also a need for further studies to investigate non-pharmacological treatments such as electrical spinal-cord stimulation, that may be considered if drug treatment fails.[28]

References

1. Shaw JE, Zimmet PZ. The epidemiology of diabetic neuropathy. *Diabetes Revs* 1999; **7**: 245–52.

2. Tesfaye S, Stephens L, Stephenson J *et al.* The prevalence of diabetic neuropathy and its relation to glycaemic control and potential risk factors: the EURODIAB IDDM Complications Study. *Diabetologia* 1996; **39**: 1377–84.

3. Tesfaye S, Chaturvedi N, Eaton SEM *et al.* Vascular risk factors and diabetic neuropathy. *New Engl J Med* 2005; **352**: 341–50.

4. Quattrini C, Tesfaye S. Understanding the impact of painful diabetic neuropathy. *Diabetes Metab Res Rev* 2003; **19**: S2–S8.

5. Jensen TS, Backonja MM, Hernandez Jimenez S *et al.* New perspectives on the management of diabetic peripheral neuropathic pain. *Diab Vasc Dis Res* 2006; **3**: 108–19.

6. Tesfaye S, Malik R, Harris N *et al.* Arterio-venous shunting and proliferating new vessels in acute painful neuropathy of rapid glycaemic control (insulin neuritis). *Diabetologia* 1996; **39**: 329–35.

7. Tesfaye S, Kempler P. Painful diabetic neuropathy. *Diabetologia* 2005; **48**: 805–7.

8. Eaton SE, Harris ND, Ibrahim S *et al.* Increased sural nerve epineurial blood flow in human subjects with painful diabetic neuropathy. *Diabetologia* 2003; **46**: 934–9.

9. Sorensen L, Molyneaux L, Yue DK. The relationship among pain, sensory loss, and small nerve fibers in diabetes. *Diabetes Care* 2006; **29**: 883–7.

10. Eaton S, Harris ND, Rajbhandari SM *et al.* Spinal cord involvement in diabetic peripheral neuropathy. *Lancet* 2001; **358**: 35–6.

11. Selvarajah D, Wilkinson ID, Emery CJ *et al.* Early involvement of the spinal cord in diabetic peripheral neuropathy. *Diabetes Care* 2006; **29**: 2664–9.

12. Dejong RN. CNS manifestations of diabetes mellitus. *Postgrad Med* 1977; **61**: 101–7.

13. Suzuki C, Ozaki I, Taosaki M *et al.* Peripheral and central conduction abnormalities in diabetes mellitus. *Neurology* 2000; **54**: 1932–7.

14. Selvarajah D, Wilkinson ID, Emery CJ *et al.* Significant correlations between neurophysiological assessments and markers of thalamic sensory neuronal dysfunction in diabetic peripheral neuropathy. *Diabetic Med* 2006; **23**(Suppl 2): A89.

15. Max MB, Lynch SA, Muir J *et al.* Effects of desipramine, amitriptyline, and fluoxetine on pain in diabetic neuropathy. *N Engl J Med* 1992; **326**: 1250–6.

16. Ray WA, Meredith S, Thapa PB *et al.* Cyclic antidepressants and the risk of sudden cardiac death. *Clin Pharmacol Ther* 2004; **75**: 234–41.

17. Goldstein DJ, Lu Y, Detke MJ *et al.* Duloxetine vs. placebo in patients with painful diabetic neuropathy. *Pain* 2005; **116**: 109–18.

18. Rowbotham MC, Goli V, Kunz NR, Lei D. Venlafaxine extended release in the treatment of painful diabetic neuropathy: a double-blind, placebo-controlled study. *Pain* 2004; **110**: 697–706.

19. Backonja M, Beydoun A, Edwards KR *et al.* Gabapentin for the symptomatic relief of painful neuropathy in patients with diabetes mellitus: a randomized controlled trial. *JAMA* 1998; **280**: 831–6.

20. Griesing T, Freeman R, Rosenstock J *et al.* Efficacy, safety, and tolerability of pregabalin treatment for diabetic peripheral neuropathy: findings from 6 randomized controlled trials. *Diabetologia* 2005; **48**(Suppl 1): A351.

21. Baillie JK, Power I, Tesfaye S *et al.* Morphine, gabapentin or their combination for neuropathic pain. *N Engl J Med* 2005; **352**: 2650–1.

22. Gilron I, Bailey JM, Tu D *et al.* Morphine, gabapentin, or their combination for neuropathic pain. *N Engl J Med* 2005; **352**: 1324–34.

23. Rauck RL, Shaibani A, Biton V *et al.* Lacosamide in painful diabetic peripheral neuropathy: a phase 2 double-blind placebo-controlled study. *Clin J Pain* 2007; **23**: 150–8.

24. Ziegler D, Nowak H, Kempler P *et al.* Treatment of symptomatic diabetic polyneuropathy with the antioxidant alpha-lipoic acid: a meta-analysis. *Diabetic Med* 2004; **21**: 114–21.

25. Ziegler D, Ametov A, Barinov A *et al.* Oral treatment with α-lipoic acid improves symptomatic diabetic polyneuropathy: The SYDNEY 2 trial. *Diabetes Care* 2006; **29**: 2365–70.

26. Finnerup NB, Otto M, McQuay HJ *et al.* Algorithm for neuropathic pain treatment: an evidence based proposal. *Pain* 2005; **118**: 289–305.

27. Daousi C, MacFarlane IA, Woodward A *et al.* Chronic painful peripheral neuropathy in an urban community: a controlled comparison of people with and without diabetes. *Diabet Med* 2004; **21**: 976–82.

28. Tesfaye S, Watt J, Benbow SJ *et al.* Electrical spinal cord stimulation for painful diabetic peripheral neuropathy. *Lancet* 1996; **348**: 1696–701.

Anaemia and renal disease in diabetes

Dr Stephen Thomas

Key points

- Test for anaemia related to kidney failure at estimated glomerular filtration rate (<60 ml/min/1.73m^2) if not earlier.
- The main benefits of anaemia treatment relate to quality of life and physical capacity.
- Ensuring adequate iron stores and use of erythropoiesis stimulating agents are both necessary for the effective treatment of kidney disease-related anaemia.
- Anaemia services need to be well coordinated.

Introduction

The World Health Organisation (WHO) defines anaemia as a haemoglobin (Hb) level <12 g/dl in pre-menopausal females, and <13 g/dl in adult males and post-menopausal females. Interest in anaemia in diabetic kidney disease has increased rapidly since it was reported that, in patients with diabetes and advanced kidney failure, anaemia is more severe and may occur at an earlier stage of kidney disease than with non diabetic glomerular disease.[1]

Fifteen cases of anaemia were described in patients with type 1 diabetes with 'early' kidney disease, stage 1 or stage 2 [estimated glomerular filtration rate (eGFR) ≥60 ml/min/1.73 m^2].[2] In a comparison of 27 patients with type 1 diabetes and diabetic kidney disease with 26 non-diabetic patients with glomerulonephritis (matched for serum creatinine ≤180 μmol/l), 13 patients with diabetes had anaemia compared with none in the non-diabetic group.[3] In type 1 diabetes, the prevalence of anaemia is 52% in patients with macroalbuminuria, 24% in patients with microalbuminuria and <8% of normoalbuminuric patients.[4]

In one small, hospital-based study, the sample prevalence of anaemia in patients with 'early' diabetic kidney disease (presence of at least microalbuminuria and serum creatinine <150 μmol/l) was 15%, all with low erythropoietin levels. Those with anaemia had a mean serum creatinine of 93 μmol/l and a median urinary albumin excretion of 46 μg/min. Prevalence of type 1 diabetes, female gender (73%) and lower creatinine clearances (57 ml/min in those with anaemia compared with 103.5 ml/min in those with normal Hb) carried higher risks of having erythropoietin-deficiency anaemia.[1]

In a cross-sectional survey of 820 patients with diabetes, approximately a quarter of patients (190 patients, 23%) had unrecognised anaemia by WHO criteria of Hb level <12 g/dl in pre-menopausal females, and <13 g/dl in adult males and post-menopausal females.[5] This prevalence of anaemia in patients with diabetes is two to three times higher than that reported for patients with similar levels of non diabetic kidney damage.

Pathogenesis of anaemia in kidney disease in diabetes

In all kidney disease, including diabetes, Hb levels fall with decreasing GFR, largely due to diminishing erythropoietin production (Figure 1).[1]

Figure 1: Haemoglobin level correlates with creatinine clearance in diabetic kidney disease.

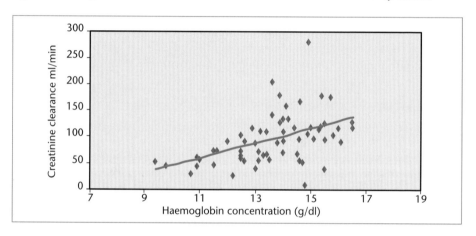

GFR is an independent predictor of Hb level, Hb being significantly lower in those with GFR <70 ml/min/1.73 m^2 compared with those with GFR 80–100 ml/min/1.73 m^2.[5] Indeed GFR >80 ml/min/1.73 m^2 may not be significantly associated with anaemia in patients without diabetes.[6]

In type 2 diabetes, patients with eGFR 60–90 ml/min/1.73 m^2 are approximately twice as likely to have anaemia as those with GFR >90 ml/min/1.73 m^2. Thus, falling GFR is the best predictor of the likelihood of anaemia in diabetic as well as in non-diabetic kidney disease.[7]

However, why anaemia may develop at higher GFR in diabetes is less clear. As in non-diabetic kidney disease, failure of erythropoietin production is central to the development of anaemia (Figure 2). Erythropoietin levels are inappropriately low and do not rise adequately with increasing severity of anaemia, in particular, in iron deficiency anaemia.[3]

Figure 2: Poor erythropoietin response to anaemia in patients with 'early' diabetic kidney disease.[3]

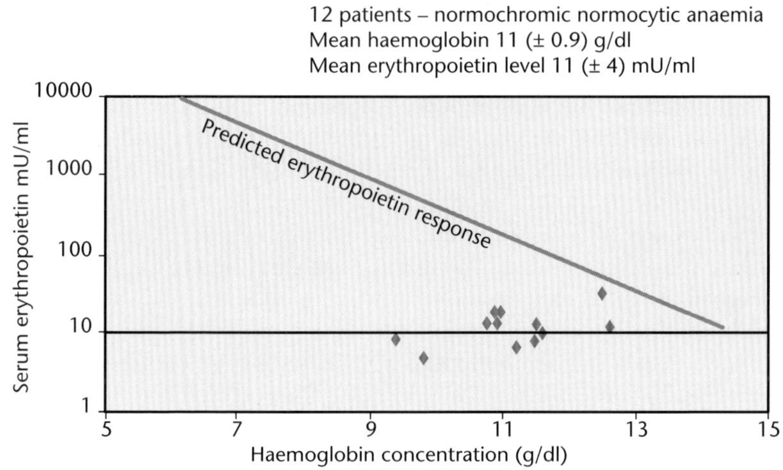

12 patients – normochromic normocytic anaemia
Mean haemoglobin 11 (± 0.9) g/dl
Mean erythropoietin level 11 (± 4) mU/ml

This failure of erythropoietin production and subsequent development of 'early' anaemia is more common in patients with type 1 diabetes, particularly females, and is not caused as a result of reduced iron stores.[8] Co-existent autonomic neuropathy may be an important factor[9] as release of erythropoietin is modulated by the sympathetic nervous system and erythropoietin-deficiency anaemia is seen in other conditions with autonomic neuropathy, particularly affecting sympathetic function.[10,11] Urinary erythropoietin losses, interstitial fibrosis (up to 90% of erythropoietin is produced by the peri-tubular fibroblasts of the kidneys) and angiotensin-converting enzyme inhibition are also possible contributors. To date, it is not known whether hyperglycaemia or high urine glucose concentrations may be relevant to the development of anaemia.

The prevalence of anaemia in people with diabetes is increased at all levels of diabetic kidney disease, even when GFR is 'well preserved'. In non-diabetic kidney disease, significant anaemia related to the kidney disease, is unlikely at GFR >60 ml/min/1.73 m^2, hence the recommendations from the renal National Service Framework to screen for anaemia in stage 3 kidney disease (eGFR 30–60 ml/min/1.73 m^2). In diabetes, this cut-off of <60 ml/min/1.73 m^2 would identify 85% of cases of anaemia in diabetic kidney disease[12] although it may be prudent to consider anaemia in symptomatic individuals with evidence of any stage of diabetic kidney disease, particularly in type 1 diabetes and in females.

Treatment of renal anaemia

The development and clinical introduction of recombinant erythropoietin therapy in the 1980s reinvigorated anaemia management in chronic kidney disease (CKD). This has been largely developed within renal units and, until recently, has been predominantly focused upon patients on renal-replacement therapy. The twin 'explosion' in the prevalence and detection of anaemia related to both diabetes and kidney disease, driven by population changes and increased screening, means demand for renal anaemia services are likely to be excessive. Furthermore, for some the need for referral to renal services may be solely related to anaemia management. These individuals are likely to have other co-morbidities and this approach may lead to fragmented care with multiple appointments. It may, therefore, be desirable for some services that anaemia management occurs in non-renal settings particularly for those with stage 3 or earlier kidney disease. As a result, the National Collaborating Centre For Chronic Conditions on behalf of the National Institute for Health and Clinical Excellence (NICE) and the Royal College Of Physicians has developed guidance on the management of anaemia in CKD of relevance for both renal units and those caring for patients with kidney disease in non-renal settings.[13] The guidance is not specific to diabetes but is for patients with diabetes and associated kidney disease and anaemia. Many of the studies performed to date have focused on patients with end stage kidney failure and some extrapolation is required for patients with earlier kidney disease who may form the bulk of new treatments in the future.

Who to treat and why?

A number of small studies have investigated the benefits of treating anaemia in patients with diabetic kidney disease (Table 1). [2,11,14–17]

Table 1: Reported benefits of treating anaemia on diabetes-specific end-points.

Beneficial effect	Total number treated	Duration	Study
Quality of life	6	12 weeks	Rarick et al. (1998)[14]
	5	12 weeks	Winkler et al. (1999)[2]
	4	6 months	Winkler et al. (2000)[15]
	172	15 months	Ritz et al. (2007)[17]
Orthostatic hypotension	4	10 weeks	Hoeldtke et al. (1993)[11]
	4	2 months	Winkler et al. (2000)[15]
Macular oedema	5	1 year	Friedman et al. (1995)[16]

Treatment with recombinant human erythropoietin over 12 weeks normalised haematocrit levels in six patients with type 1 diabetes and unexplained symptomatic anaemia with serum creatinine <177 μmol/l, with associated improvement in quality of life.[14]

In five patients with type 1 diabetes and renal anaemia, recombinant erythropoietin therapy increased Hb concentration with a corresponding improvement in patient 'well-being'.[2] Hoeldtke and Streeten treated eight patients with orthostatic hypotension, four of whom had type 1 diabetes and autonomic neuropathy, with recombinant erythropoietin therapy, resulting in increases in standing systolic and diastolic blood pressure after treatment for 6–10 weeks, with improvements in orthostatic dizziness in six of the patients.[11] The increase in standing systolic blood pressure following treatment with recombinant erythropoietin was also shown in a study of four female patients with orthostatic hypotension, erythropoietin-deficiency anaemia and diabetic autonomic neuropathy.[15] After withdrawal of erythropoietin, systolic blood pressure declined, suggesting that the increase in blood pressure was dependent on the Hb concentration. Finally, a very small study of five patients found that diabetic macular oedema improved following erythropoietin treatment for 1 year in patients with renal insufficiency;[16] the authors suggested that the improvement in oedema might have resulted from reduced tissue and cellular hypoxia following anaemia treatment.

It has long been postulated that treating anaemia has a positive impact on mortality. This seems likely but at what level of Hb this benefit would operate is less clear and whether correcting the 'moderate' anaemia seen in earlier kidney disease would impart this benefit is uncertain. Data suggest that anaemia is an independent predictor of left ventricular hypertrophy in patients with CKD and small intervention studies have shown that raising haematocrit by approximately 25% reduces left ventricular mass index.[18] In addition, cross-sectional studies found an increased mortality in those with Hb <11g/dl compared to those with Hb of between 11 and 13 g/dl.[19]

Intervention studies to date, however, have not been supportive of aggressive normalisation of Hb concentrations. Besarab and colleagues examined the risks and benefits of treatment to maintain a normal (42%) compared with a low (30%) haematocrit for 14 months in 1,233 patients (~56% with diabetes), with clinical evidence of congestive heart failure or ischaemic heart disease undergoing haemodialysis.[20] The study was terminated early when there were excess deaths among the patients in the normal-haematocrit group [risk ratio for the normal-haematocrit group vs. the low-haematocrit group 1.3; 95% confidence interval (CI): 0.9–1.9]. The CHOIR study, published in 2006, treated 1,432 patients with CKD, ~50% of whom had diabetes, with recombinant erythropoietin. In total, 715 patients were randomised to achieve target Hb of 13.5 g/dl and 717 randomised to 11.3 g/dl – slightly strange targets as they were amended during the trial.[21] Patients treated to the higher Hb level suffered more from the primary end-point of death, myocardial infarction, hospitalisation for congestive heart failure, and stroke, with a hazard ratio of 1.34 (95% CI: 1.03–1.74) compared with those treated to lower Hb levels. There were no discernible benefits seen in those treated to the higher target.

The CREATE study examined 603 patients with stage 4 kidney disease (eGFR 15–35 ml/min/1.73m^2) with Hb levels between 11 and 12.5 g/dl, approximately 25% of whom had diabetes.[22] In this study, correction of Hb from 13 to 15 g/dl had no discernable effect on any of the eight cardiovascular end-points. Improvements were seen in 'general health' and physical function; however, more of these patients required dialysis, and headaches and hypertensive episodes were more prevalent. The ACORD study[17] examined 172 patients with diabetes and stage 1 to stage 3 kidney disease (eGFR 30–90 ml/min/1.73 m^2), with moderate anaemia randomised to treatment to achieve target Hb of either 10.5–11.5 g/dl or 13–15 g/dl for 15 months. Patients with the higher target achieved Hb of 13.5 g/dl, but no statistical benefit was seen on left ventricular mass index. However, quality of life was improved compared with the group with a lower target, who achieved a target Hb of 12 g/dl. There was no effect on decline of kidney function between the two groups.

These studies suggest that, at best, there is no cardiovascular or renal benefit from aggressive normalisation of Hb; however, whether it increases cardiovascular morbidity/mortality or accelerates rate of kidney disease progression remains uncertain.

Parameters such as quality of life, exercise capacity and physical function do improve with treatment and potentially make it worthwhile maintaining therapy. Other postulated benefits of correction of anaemia include improved cognitive function, improved sexual function, reduced transfusion requirements, and reduced hospitalisation. However, in many of these areas there remains a paucity of literature.

How to treat?
Erythropoiesis-stimulating agents
Most individuals with significant renal anaemia will require recombinant erythropoiesis-stimulating agents (ESA). There are several commercially available preparations differing in duration of onset, frequency of injection, route of administration, and cost. Guidelines for use have generated a titration algorithm, which may be useful as a basis for therapy (Appendix 1). For most individuals, erythropoietin treatment is a self-administered subcutaneous injection via a pen device, once to twice a week.

Iron
The availability of iron is crucial for red blood cell production. Functional iron deficiency may be an important contributor to renal anaemia. This functional deficiency is a state where ferritin levels are normal but there is a lack of free iron to support red cell production, particularly when erythropoiesis is stimulated by recombinant erythropoietin therapy. This state is different to the traditional absolute iron deficiency, usually related to blood loss or poor dietary intake/absorption when iron stores are depleted, such that ferritin levels are <20 μg/l. Differentiating between the two can, at times, be complicated. Accurate assessment of functional iron deficiency – the adequacy of iron stores for

efficient effective erythropoiesis – is complex. It seems easier to define that iron stores are not abnormally high than to demonstrate that there is adequate available iron for erythropoiesis. Commonly used measures of functional iron deficiency include ferritin, transferrin saturation and percentage of hypochromic red cells.

Treatment of anaemia with recombinant erythropoietin requires adequate iron stores and an adequate supply of 'available' iron. In functional iron deficiency, absorption of dietary iron, and even supplemented oral iron, may be poor. In diabetes, this may be compounded by associated diabetic gut disease. Some individuals will have an impressive rise in Hb purely by supplementing iron, usually intravenously. It is, therefore, important that all iron deficiency, functional or absolute, is treated prior to and during erythropoietin therapy.

Parenteral iron is, therefore, the treatment of choice for functional iron deficiency. The introduction of ferric sodium gluconate and iron saccharate has significantly reduced the risk of life-threatening allergic reactions, but there are some concerns that they may predispose to infection, and therefore should be avoided during active bacterial infections, such as infected diabetic foot ulceration.

Practicalities of treatment

Management of anaemia is complex. To maintain Hb levels in the desirable range requires timely adjustment of ESA dose and iron administration. Failure to do so may result in costly, ineffective treatment or 'undesirably high' Hb levels. NICE guidelines give advice on the 'aspirational range', rather than target level, of Hb and advice on when dose-adjustment is required to reduce over- or under-shooting (Appendix 1). Patient education and support is of great importance, as are arrangements between prescribers and maintenance of supply to patients. This should not be foreign to diabetes services as similarities already exist with arrangements for insulin and growth-hormone replacement.

Conventionally, each unit wishing to develop anaemia services will have anaemia specialist nurses/coordinators, although other models do exist. There is also the national Anaemia Nurse Specialist Association. In some areas, anaemia management is being set up in primary care in a similar way to insulin management.

Conclusion

Anaemia is an increasingly recognised association of diabetes, mostly related to the development of kidney disease and possibly occurring at an earlier stage of kidney failure in those with diabetes. Effective treatment is available and the benefits and rationale for treatment are increasingly well understood. Testing for anaemia in at-risk individuals and having effective treatment protocols and systems should form an integral part of diabetes care.

Appendix 1: NICE guideline on management of anaemia in chronic kidney disease.[13]

Key messages from guideline

- Management of anaemia should be considered in people with anaemia of CKD

- CKD when the Hb level is ≤11g/dl

- Treatment with ESA should be offered to patients with anaemia of CKD who are likely to benefit in terms of quality of life and physical function

- ESA therapy should be clinically effective, consistent and safe in people with anaemia of CKD

- To achieve this, the prescriber and patient should agree a plan which is patient-centred and includes:
  - Continuity of drug supply
  - Flexibility of where the drug is delivered and administered
  - Lifestyle and preferences of the patient
  - Cost of drug supply
  - Desire for self-care where appropriate
  - Regular review of the plan in light of changing needs

- In people with anaemia of CKD, treatment should maintain stable Hb levels between 10.5 g/dl and 12.5 g/dl for adults. This should be achieved by:
  - Considering adjustments to treatment, typically when Hb rises above 12.0 g/dl or falls below 11.0 g/dl
  - Taking patient preferences, symptoms and co-morbidity into account and revising the aspirational range and action thresholds accordingly

- Age alone should not be a determinant for treatment of anaemia of CKD

- People receiving ESA maintenance therapy should be given iron supplements to keep their serum ferritin between 200 µg/l and 500 µg/l in both haemodialysis patients and non-haemodialysis patients, and either
  - The transferrin saturation level above 20% (unless ferritin >800 µg/l) or
  - Percentage hypochromic red cells <6% (unless ferritin >800 ug/l)

- In practice it is likely this will require intravenous iron

References

1. Thomas S, Rampersad M. Anaemia in diabetes. *Acta Diabetol* 2004; **41** (Suppl 1): S13–7.

2. Winkler AS, Marsden J, Chaudhuri KR *et al.* Erythropoietin depletion and anaemia in diabetes mellitus. *Diabet Med* 1999; **16**: 813–9.

3. Bosman DR, Winkler AS, Marsden JT *et al.* Anemia with erythropoietin deficiency occurs early in diabetic nephropathy. *Diabetes Care* 2001; **24**: 495–9.

4. Thomas MC, MacIsaac RJ, Tsalamandris C *et al.* Anemia in patients with type 1 diabetes. *J Clin Endocrinol Metab* 2004; **89**: 4359–63.

5. Thomas MC, MacIsaac RJ, Tsalamandris C *et al.* Unrecognized anemia in patients with diabetes: a cross-sectional survey. *Diabetes Care* 2003; **26**: 1164–9.

6. Kazmi WH, Kausz AT, Khan S *et al.* Anemia: an early complication of chronic renal insufficiency. *Am J Kidney Dis* 2001; **38**: 803–12.

7. Thomas MC, Tsalamandris C, MacIsaac RJ, Jerums G. The epidemiology of hemoglobin levels in patients with type 2 diabetes. *Am J Kidney Dis* 2006; **48**: 537–45.

8. Rampersad MTS. Erythropoietin deficiency anaemia is common in early diabetic kidney disease. *Diabet Med* 2002; **19** (Suppl. 2).

9. Bosman DR, Osborne CA, Marsden JT *et al.* Erythropoietin response to hypoxia in patients with diabetic autonomic neuropathy and non-diabetic chronic renal failure. *Diabet Med* 2002; **19**: 65–9.

10. Ghirlanda G, Cotroneo P, Todaro L *et al.* Erythropoietin depletion and anaemia in diabetes mellitus. *Diabet Med* 2000; **17**: 410.

11. Hoeldtke RD, Streeten DH. Treatment of orthostatic hypotension with erythropoietin. *N Engl J Med* 1993; **329**: 611–5.

12. Al-Khoury S, Afzali B, Shah N *et al.* Anaemia in diabetic patients with chronic kidney disease-prevalence and predictors. *Diabetologia* 2006; **49**: 1183–9.

13. Anaemia Management in Chronic Kidney Disease: National Clinical Guideline For Management in Adults and Children. NICE Clinical Guidelines. 2007.

14. Rarick MU, Espina BM, Colley DT *et al.* Treatment of a unique anemia in patients with IDDM with epoetin alfa. *Diabetes Care* 1998; **21**: 423–6.

15. Winkler AS, Watkins PJ. Long-term treatment of the anaemia in Type 1 diabetes mellitus with erythropoietin. *Diabet Med* 2000; **17**: 250–1.

16. Friedman EA, Brown CD, Berman DH. Erythropoietin in diabetic macular edema and renal insufficiency. *Am J Kidney Dis* 1995; **26**: 202–8.

17. Ritz E, Laville M, Bilous RW *et al.* Target level for hemoglobin correction in patients with diabetes and CKD: primary results of the Anemia Correction in Diabetes (ACORD) Study. *Am J Kidney Dis* 2007; **49**: 194–207.

18. Hayashi T, Suzuki A, Shoji T *et al.* Cardiovascular effect of normalizing the hematocrit level during erythropoietin therapy in predialysis patients with chronic renal failure. *Am J Kidney Dis* 2000; **35**: 250–6.

19. Wolfe RA, Hulbert-Shearon TE, Ashby VB *et al.* Improvements in dialysis patient mortality are associated with improvements in urea reduction ratio and hematocrit, 1999 to 2002. *Am J Kidney Dis* 2005; **45**: 127–35.

20. Besarab A, Bolton WK, Browne JK *et al.* The effects of normal as compared with low hematocrit values in patients with cardiac disease who are receiving hemodialysis and epoetin. *N Engl J Med* 1998; **339**: 584–90.

21. Singh AK, Szczech L, Tang KL *et al.* Correction of anemia with epoetin alfa in chronic kidney disease. *N Engl J Med* 2006; **355**: 2085–98.

22. Drueke TB, Locatelli F, Clyne N *et al.* Normalization of hemoglobin level in patients with chronic kidney disease and anemia. *N Engl J Med* 2006; **355**: 2071–84.

Non-alcoholic fatty liver disease and diabetes: clinical implications and management

Professor Christopher D Byrne, Dr Sarah H Wild

Key points

- The exact prevalence of non-alcoholic fatty liver disease (NAFLD) in diabetes is uncertain but is probably at least 75% of patients with type 2 diabetes.
- Liver ultrasound only identifies liver fat and not liver inflammation in NAFLD.
- Non-alcoholic steatohepatitis (NASH) is associated with progression over time and a worse cardiovascular outcome.
- Biochemical markers lack sensitivity and specificity to identify NAFLD, but new algorithms are currently being developed and tested that may be useful in the near future.
- Pioglitazone and rosiglitazone are showing promise in research studies as unlicensed new treatments for NAFLD.

Definition and prevalence of NAFLD

Non-alcoholic fatty liver disease (NAFLD) is emerging as the most common chronic liver condition in the Western world. NAFLD is associated with insulin resistance and increasingly occurs in the cluster of features of the metabolic syndrome (Figure 1). NAFLD is a risk factor for cardiovascular disease (CVD), independent of other features of the metabolic syndrome and conventional cardiovascular risk factors. The precise pathogenesis of NAFLD is unclear and although hepatic fat accumulation is required, in some individuals this does not progress to the more severe forms of NAFLD, suggesting that some product of lipid metabolism 'triggers' the inflammatory and fibrotic pathways.

Figure 1: Schematic figure showing NAFLD as a newer feature of the metabolic syndrome.

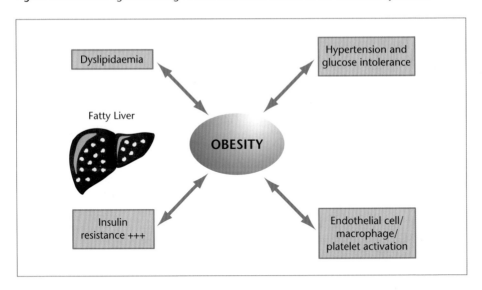

Abnormal liver function tests (LFTs) are highly prevalent in type 2 diabetes and it has been estimated that 75% of patients with type 2 diabetes may have some form of NAFLD, which may progress to end-stage liver disease. NAFLD is now considered to be the hepatic component of the metabolic syndrome[1] and although the characteristic histology resembles that of alcohol-induced liver injury, NAFLD occurs in individuals who consume little alcohol (<10 g per day).

NAFLD refers to a wide spectrum of liver damage, ranging from simple steatosis to steatohepatitis, advanced fibrosis and cirrhosis. Figure 2 (A–C) shows the typical features of steatohepatitis. In this biopsy sample from a patient with NAFLD, the architecture is preserved but there is significant perivenular, pericellular, sinusoidal fibrosis (Figure 2C). No fibrotic bridging to portal tracts is evident and the scar tissue is mature. There is grade 3 fatty infiltration with several ballooned hepatocytes and many vacuolated nuclei (Figure 2A). Grade 2 haemosiderosis is also evident (Figure 2B). These appearances are those of steatohepatitis and, in the absence of alcohol, are consistent with a moderately severe staging of NAFLD i.e. non-alcoholic steatohepatitis (NASH).

NAFLD is regarded as the most common cause of increased liver enzymes in the USA, associated with type 2 diabetes, obesity and hyperlipidemia. The reported prevalence of obesity with NAFLD varies between 30% and 100%. The prevalence of NAFLD in type 2 diabetes varies between 10% and 75%, and hyperlipidemia between 20 and 92%.[1] There are few studies of the natural history of NAFLD but a recent study by Adams *et al*, of 420 patients diagnosed with NAFLD who were followed up between 1980 and 2000, showed that survival was lower in patients with NAFLD than the expected survival for the general population because of CVD and malignancy.[2]

Figure 2: Typical features of steatohepatitis. No fibrotic bridging to portal tracts is evident and the scar tissue is mature. These appearances are those of steatohepatitis and in the absence of alcohol these findings were consistent with a moderately severe form of NAFLD, i.e. NASH.

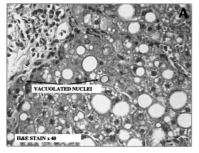

A: In this biopsy sample from a patient with NAFLD, the architecture is preserved and there is grade 3 fatty infiltration with several ballooned hepatocytes and many vacuolated nuclei.

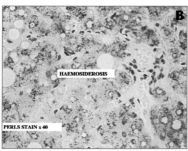

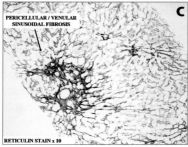

B: There is evidence of Grade 2 haemosiderosis as shown by the PERLS stain and

C: marked perivenular, pericellular, sinusoidal fibrosis as shown by the reticulin stain.

The prevalence of diabetes was 22%, dyslipidaemia 23%, hypertension 22% and cirrhosis 5%.

In type 2 diabetes the prevalence of NAFLD is probably much higher than among the general population and it is thought that up to 75% of patients with type 2 diabetes and 75% of patients with obesity have some form of NAFLD.[3,4] It is difficult to obtain precise estimates of the prevalence, as establishing a diagnosis is based on the results of a liver biopsy; an intrusive procedure which is inappropriate to use on large populations.

How is NAFLD diagnosed at present?

A finding of abnormal LFTs presents the clinician with several management problems:

- Does the patient need further investigation to identify the cause?
- Is a liver biopsy required?
- Is treatment with statins safe, knowing these agents adversely affect LFTs?
- Is treatment for NAFLD required?
- Is monitoring required, and if so, how?

Unfortunately to date there is no non-invasive simple test with good sensitivity and specificity to identify individuals with NAFLD that can be used. Liver ultrasound will only identify liver fat and will not help diagnose liver inflammation or fibrosis. The poor sensitivity of liver ultrasound to diagnose hepatic inflammation and fibrosis is significant as the different degrees of severity of NAFLD may indicate different natural histories for progression of liver disease.

A typical algorithm for investigating a patient with suspected NAFLD is shown in Figure 3.

Figure 3: Algorithm for investigation of NAFLD in 2007.

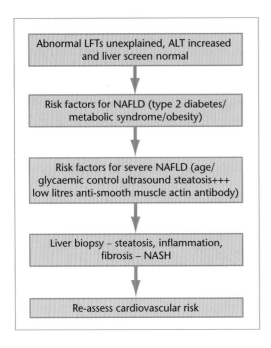

Abnormal LFTs unexplained, ALT increased and liver screen normal

↓

Risk factors for NAFLD (type 2 diabetes/ metabolic syndrome/obesity)

↓

Risk factors for severe NAFLD (age/ glycaemic control ultrasound steatosis+++ low litres anti-smooth muscle actin antibody)

↓

Liver biopsy – steatosis, inflammation, fibrosis – NASH

↓

Re-assess cardiovascular risk

The dilemma facing the clinician is which patients to refer for liver biopsy and which to monitor with non-invasive tests. To date, there is no simple answer to this dilemma and limited evidence upon which to base any recommendation regarding which patients to refer for biopsy. In practice, the patients with extensive liver steatosis, confirmed by ultrasound and alanine amino-transferase (ALT) levels >2–3x the upper limit of normal, tend to be those in whom liver biopsy is considered. Often the personal preferences of the hepatologist to whom the patient is referred dictate which patients are further investigated by liver biopsy.

The natural history of NAFLD and associations between NAFLD and CVD

Although NAFLD is part of the metabolic syndrome, it has recently been recognised as an independent risk marker for CVD,[5–7] perhaps reflecting the fact that NAFLD comprises a spectrum of liver conditions, including fat accumulation, inflammation and fibrosis of varying severity. Moreover, overweight, smoking and diabetes are independent predictors of hepatic fibrosis.[8] The presence of which, along with hepatic inflammation, can contribute to progression of NAFLD chronic liver disease (CLD), an important cause of death in the UK.

The largest study to describe the natural history of NAFLD has recently reported the results of a 13.7-year mean follow-up of patients with biopsy-proven NAFLD.[9] One of the main findings of this landmark study, undertaken in relatively young individuals (mean age 47 years at diagnosis), was that survival was reduced by 10% (compared to a general age-matched population) in patients with NASH. Furthermore, this study confirmed that there is marked variability in outcome for patients with different forms of NAFLD as in contrast to those people with NASH, mortality was unaffected in patients with simple steatosis. Therefore, the evidence emphasises that NAFLD represents a heterogeneous cluster of liver pathologies associated with variable risk that require a more precise diagnosis as the evidence suggests that patients with NASH are at greater risk than those people with only steatosis. Importantly, the study shows a differential impact on cardiovascular outcome and future survival, according to the histological type of NAFLD at initial diagnosis. For example, 41% of patients with evidence of fibrosis in the initial biopsy showed evidence of worsening liver fibrosis over time. Patients with NASH, (those with inflammation and fibrosis) present in the initial biopsy, had increased mortality over time compared with those with a more benign form of NAFLD (steatosis alone) at original histological diagnosis. There was a 14-fold increase in deaths directly attributable to liver disease in patients with an initial diagnosis of NASH compared with the control population without NAFLD. Importantly, over the 13.7-year follow-up, increased mortality was also related to cardiovascular death. Thus for the first time, we have convincing evidence that there is a pressing need to diagnose NAFLD and to identify the more severe sub-group of NAFLD.

The initial severity of NAFLD may be associated with different degrees of risk for CVD. Recent data also suggest that NAFLD may be an important novel cardiovascular risk factor in type 2 diabetes[10,11] even after adjusting for conventional cardiovascular risk factors and for other standard features of the metabolic syndrome. In recent data by Targher *et al*, type 2 diabetes patients (n = 2,839) had an unadjusted prevalence of NAFLD of 69.5%, and NAFLD was the most common cause (81.5%) of hepatic steatosis on ultrasound.[12] The prevalence of NAFLD increased with age (65.4% among participants aged 40–59 years and 74.6% among those aged ≥60 years; p <0.001) with an age-adjusted prevalence of 71.1% in men and 68% in women. NAFLD patients had a higher age (p<0.001), and sex-adjusted prevalence of coronary (26.6% vs. 18.3%), cerebrovascular (20.0 vs. 13.3%) and peripheral (15.4 vs. 10.0%) vascular disease than their counterparts without NAFLD. In logistic regression analysis, NAFLD was associated with prevalent CVD, independent of classical risk factors, glycaemic control, medications and features of the metabolic syndrome.[12]

Risk prediction for cardiovascular events in type 2 diabetes is poor and may be underestimated by a third.[13] It is hugely variable with an almost five-fold increased risk of coronary heart disease death, if patients have all five US National Cholesterol Education Program ATPIII metabolic syndrome features, compared with having only one feature (i.e. hyperglycaemia).[14] Given this marked heterogeneity of cardiovascular risk,[14] we have shown that patients with NAFLD and obesity are markedly more insulin resistant than those with obesity alone.[15] Increased clearance of cortisol was also present in these people.[16] It is uncertain whether the marked insulin resistance with NAFLD explains the additional increase in CVD in a subgroup of people with type 2 diabetes. It is plausible that diagnosing the more severe forms of NAFLD in type 2 diabetes may identify a subgroup of people at very high risk of CVD that need particularly aggressive intervention.

Hepatic fat accumulation and inflammation are key, early features of NAFLD.[1,17] If the disease progresses to CLD[18] with cirrhosis, there is a further burden to the individual and to the health service. Importantly, it is now recognised that diabetes is associated with an approximately two- to three-fold increased risk of cirrhosis and a recent review has estimated that the prevalence of diabetes in 'cryptogenic' cirrhosis is around 40%,[19] suggesting that patients may have originally had NAFLD that progressed over time.

Non-invasive diagnosis of NAFLD in the near future

Abnormal LFT results are an imperfect measure of NAFLD, and although simple hepatic steatosis can be diagnosed by liver ultrasound, liver biopsy is the current reference standard for diagnosis and monitoring of NAFLD. Liver biopsy is invasive, costly and has a risk of morbidity and even mortality.[20–22] Moreover, the precision of the diagnosis is affected by tissue sampling and by inter-observer variation between pathologists. The utility of non-invasive serum markers associated with liver fibrosis in NAFLD has recently been reviewed.[23] A panel of markers has been developed that have 84% sensitivity and 91% specificity for detecting moderate to severe fibrosis (equivalent to liver biopsy Ishak 4–6 staging) in NAFLD.[24]

From this work, the European Liver Fibrosis (ELF) score was developed as a result of the international multicentre cohort study, and serum marker concentrations were compared with fibrosis stage in liver biopsy specimens obtained from 1021 subjects. Discriminant analysis was used to identify an algorithm that combined age, hyaluronic acid, amino-terminal propeptide of type III collagen and tissue inhibitor of matrix metalloproteinase 1 to derive the ELF score. This algorithm was then evaluated using a validation set of biopsy specimens and serum samples and the derived score found to be useful in detecting moderate-to-severe NAFLD (equivalent to liver biopsy Ishak staging 4–6). It is this form of NAFLD that it is important to identify, because as discussed, this is the form that is most likely to progress and that is associated with a worse cardiovascular outcome. Moreover, in the largest follow-up study of NAFLD,[9] the authors concluded that they were not able to find simple clinical parameters that could predict progression of liver fibrosis in people with a diagnosis of NAFLD at baseline.

Thus, in patients with diabetes there is a pressing need to have simple non-invasive diagnostic markers that:

- Can be used to identify the more severe forms of NAFLD
- Can be used to monitor progression of liver disease
- Can be used to test the effects of new agents to treat NAFLD, without resorting to liver biopsy.

What is the pathogenesis of hepatic damage in NASH?

Currently, insulin resistance appears to be the main axis in the production of NASH. An increased fatty acid supply to the liver increases resistance to the antilypolytic action of insulin, although the exact molecular and hormonal mechanism of insulin resistance is not known. Several molecular targets are thought to be involved in inhibiting the actions of insulin. These include plasma cell-1 (a membrane glycoprotein that has a role in insulin resistance, reducing insulin-stimulated tyrosine kinase activity) and adiponectin, a protein secreted from adipose tissue which decreases hyperglycaemia, reverses insulin resistance and causes sustained weight loss, without affecting food intake in an animal model of NASH. As a potential role for tumour necrosis factor α has been proposed in the development of NASH, such a cytokine might be considered as a common link between insulin resistance and NASH, especially in subjects with obesity and/or type 2 diabetes.

Hepatic lipid metabolism in NAFLD

Sterol-regulatory element-binding proteins

Sterol-regulatory element-binding proteins (SREBPs) are key transcription factors that regulate hepatocyte–lipid homeostasis and may be important in the pathogenesis of NAFLD. The mammalian genome encodes three SREBP isoforms, designated SREBP-1a, SREBP-1c and SREBP-2. The promoter of the *SREBP-1c* gene contains response elements for insulin and glucagon, as well as liver X-activated receptors.

Overexpression of SREBP-1c in the liver of transgenic mice produces a triglyceride-enriched fatty liver with no increase in cholesterol, while SREBP-2 overexpression in transgenic mice resulted in a 28-fold increase in cholesterol synthesis.[25] In the livers of knockout mice that lack expression of all SREBPs, there is a marked decrease in the insulin-induced stimulation of lipogenic gene expression.[25] Furthermore, SREBP-1c may also contribute to the regulation of glucose uptake and glucose synthesis through induction of expression of glucokinase, a key enzyme in glucose utilisation. Fatty liver of insulin resistance is caused by SREBP-1c, which is elevated in response to the high insulin levels. Thus, SREBP-1c may play a crucial role in regulation of hepatic glucose and triglyceride, which are two major factors involved in the pathogenesis of NAFLD.

Hepatic fat accumulation and inflammation

A key transcription factor complex involved in inflammation is nuclear factor-kappa B (NFκB). In fat-laden hepatocytes, NFκB upregulates synthesis of anti-apoptotic bcl-2 that prevents release of cytochrome C from mitochondria. NFκB also increases transcription of protective enzymes such as inducible nitric oxide synthase which prevents activation of apoptotic caspases such as caspase 3. It has been suggested that the vulnerability of fat-laden hepatocytes is mainly due to reduced adenosine triphosphate content which may be due to decreased mitochondrial oxidative capacity and/or associated overexpression of uncoupling protein 2.

The liver has a large amount of macrophages (Kupffer) cells, and these cells have considerable potential to produce cytokines, prostanoids, and reactive oxygen species (ROS). ROS and superoxide that are not scavenged by macrophages will produce lipid peroxides, potentially producing further hepatic damage, the net consequence of which is severe fibrosis, cirrhosis and end-stage liver disease.

How should we treat NAFLD?

Currently, there is no definitive treatment for NAFLD. Good metabolic control is recommended in patients with diabetes or hyperlipidaemia, but it is not a curative treatment. The aim of a treatment should be to reverse the progression of NAFLD and to prevent liver-related illness and death.

Many people with type 2 diabetes are now prescribed statins but to date there are limited data testing the efficacy of treatment on NAFLD. The evidence suggests that statins are probably safe in most people with NAFLD but more data are needed. Both weight loss and exercise improve insulin sensitivity and the current evidence suggests that gradual weight loss should be advocated in all patients with NAFLD, as the majority of subjects are overweight. However, to date there is no randomised controlled trial evidence demonstrating the benefit of any lifestyle intervention in NAFLD. A reasonable target weight loss would be 10% of body weight over 6 months, as rapid weight loss should be avoided due to the risk of worsening inflammation and fibrosis.

Peroxisome proliferator-activated receptor γ agonists may prove to be useful in reducing hepatic fat in patients with NAFLD, protecting against adverse metabolic consequences and the ultimate development of cirrhosis in patients with fatty livers.[26] Recently, pioglitazone was shown not only to improve insulin sensitivity and decrease liver fat content, but also to improve histology features of NAFLD in the liver.[27] Interesting recent evidence suggests that the hepatic cannabinoid 1 receptor antagonist, rimonabant, decreases hepatic fibrogenesis in mice.[28] Whether this new therapeutic class of drug is of benefit in humans with NAFLD now needs to be tested.

Conclusion

NAFLD is most probably the hepatic manifestation of the metabolic syndrome and NAFLD is regarded as a common cause of increased ALT in type 2 diabetes.

Acknowledgements

The authors wish to thank Lucinda England for her assistance in the preparation of this chapter.

References

1. Ahmed MH, Byrne CD. Non-alcoholic steatohepatitis. In: Byrne CD, Wild SH (eds.) *The Metabolic Syndrome.* Chichester, UK: John Wiley & Sons Ltd 2005: 279–305.

2. Adams LA, Lymp JF, St Sauver J *et al.* The natural history of nonalcoholic fatty liver disease: a population-based cohort study. *Gastroenterology* 2005; **129**: 113–21.

3. Medina J, Fernandez-Salazar LI, Garcia-Buey L, Moreno-Otero R. Approach to the pathogenesis and treatment of nonalcoholic steatohepatitis. *Diabetes Care* 2004; **27**: 2057–66.

4. Farrell GC, Larter CZ. Nonalcoholic fatty liver disease: from steatosis to cirrhosis. *Hepatology* 2006; **43** (Suppl 1): S99–S112.

5. McCullough AJ. The clinical features, diagnosis and natural history of nonalcoholic fatty liver disease. *Clin Liver Dis* 2004; **8**: 521–33, viii.

6. Marchesini G, Bugianesi E, Forlani G *et al.* Nonalcoholic fatty liver, steatohepatitis, and the metabolic syndrome. *Hepatology* 2003; **37**: 917–23.

7. Cigolini M, Targher G, Agostino G *et al.* Liver steatosis and its relation to plasma haemostatic factors in apparently healthy men – role of the metabolic syndrome. *Thromb Haemost* 1996; **76**: 69–73.

8. de Lédinghen V, Ratziu V, Causse X *et al.* Diagnostic and predictive factors of significant liver fibrosis and minimal lesions in patients with persistent unexplained elevated transaminases. A prospective multicenter study. *J Hepatol* 2006; **45**: 592–9.

9. Ekstedt M, Franzen LE, Mathiesen UL *et al.* Long-term follow-up of patients with NAFLD and elevated liver enzymes. *Hepatology* 2006; **44**: 865–73.

10. Targher G, Bertolini L, Poli F *et al.* Nonalcoholic fatty liver disease and risk of future cardiovascular events among type 2 diabetic patients. *Diabetes* 2005; **54**: 3541–6.

11. Targher G, Bertolini L, Padovani R *et al.* Increased prevalence of cardiovascular disease in Type 2 diabetic patients with non-alcoholic fatty liver disease. *Diabet Med* 2006; **23**: 403–9.

12. Targher G, Bertolini L, Padovani R *et al.* Prevalence of nonalcoholic fatty liver disease and its association with cardiovascular disease among type 2 diabetic patients. *Diabetes Care* 2007; **30**: 1212–8.

13. Guzder RN, Gatling W, Mullee MA *et al.* Prognostic value of the Framingham cardiovascular risk equation and the UKPDS risk engine for coronary heart disease in newly diagnosed type 2 diabetes: results from a United Kingdom study. *Diabet Med* 2005; **22**: 554–62.

14. Guzder RN, Gatling W, Mullee MA *et al.* Impact of metabolic syndrome criteria on cardiovascular disease risk in people with newly diagnosed type 2 diabetes. *Diabetologia* 2006; **49**: 49–55.

15. Holt HB, Wild SH, Wood PJ *et al.* Non-esterified fatty acid concentrations are independently associated with hepatic steatosis in obese subjects. *Diabetologia* 2006; **49**: 141–8.

16. Holt HB, Wild SH, Postle AD *et al.* Cortisol clearance and associations with insulin sensitivity, body fat and fatty liver in middle-aged men. *Diabetologia* 2007; **50**: 1024–32.

17. Day CP, James OF. Hepatic steatosis: innocent bystander or guilty party? *Hepatology* 1998; **27**: 1463–6.

18. Angulo P. Nonalcoholic fatty liver disease. *N Engl J Med* 2002; **346**: 1221–31.

19. Maheshwari A, Thuluvath PJ. Cryptogenic cirrhosis and NAFLD: are they related? *Am J Gastroenterol* 2006; **101**: 664–8.

20. Cadranel JF, Rufat P, Degos F. Practices of liver biopsy in France: results of a prospective nationwide survey. For the Group of Epidemiology of the French Association for the Study of the Liver (AFEF). *Hepatology* 2000; **32**: 477–81.

21. Grant A, Neuberger J. Guidelines on the use of liver biopsy in clinical practice. British Society of Gastroenterology. *Gut* 1999; **45** (Suppl 4): IV1–IV11.

22. Piccinino F, Sagnelli E, Pasquale G, Giusti G. Complications following percutaneous liver biopsy. A multicentre retrospective study on 68,276 biopsies. *J Hepatol* 1986; **2**: 165–73.

23. Guha IN, Parkes J, Roderick PR *et al.* Non-invasive markers associated with liver fibrosis in non-alcoholic fatty liver disease. *Gut* 2006; **55**: 1650–60.

24. Rosenberg WM, Voelker M, Thiel R *et al.* Serum markers detect the presence of liver fibrosis: a cohort study. *Gastroenterology* 2004; **127**: 1704–13.

25. Matsuda M, Korn BS, Hammer RE *et al.* SREBP cleavage-activating protein (SCAP) is required for increased lipid synthesis in liver induced by cholesterol deprivation and insulin elevation. *Genes Dev* 2001; **15**: 1206–16.

26. Isley WL. Hepatotoxicity of thiazolidinediones. *Expert Opin Drug Saf* 2003; **2**: 581–6.

27. Belfort R, Harrison SA, Brown K *et al.* A placebo-controlled trial of pioglitazone in subjects with nonalcoholic steatohepatitis. *N Engl J Med* 2006; **355**: 2297–307.

28. Teixeira-Clerc F, Julien B, Grenard P *et al.* CB1 cannabinoid receptor antagonism: a new strategy for the treatment of liver fibrosis. *Nat Med* 2006; **12**: 671–6.

Estimated glomerular filtration rate and diabetes

Professor Rudolf Bilous

Key points

- Estimated glomerular filtration rate (eGFR) is here to stay as the basis of classification of chronic kidney disease (CKD).
- At present eGFR uses the Modification of Diet in Renal Disease (MDRD) 4 part equation with correction for standardised serum creatinine assays.
- eGFR is not a precise measure and significantly underestimates clearance derived GFR at values >90 ml/min/1.73 m². However, it is a better indicator of renal impairment than serum creatinine alone.
- eGFR may be more useful in long-term monitoring of patients by identifying those with a more rapid decline in renal function.
- Patients with values <60 ml/min/1.73 m² have CKD by definition and should be investigated for anaemia and secondary hyperparathyroidism. In addition, they should be targeted for intensive cardiovascular disease (CVD) risk factor reduction.
- Current guidelines set out criteria for referral and are outlined in this article.

What is GFR?

Glomerular filtration rate or GFR is a measure of the volume of plasma that is filtered by the renal glomeruli in unit time and is conventionally reported in ml/min.

In essence, it is an estimate of the ability of the kidneys to excrete nitrogenous waste (in humans mostly urea) that cannot be removed by any other means. GFR declines with ageing so the normal values vary but is usually given as 120 ml/min/1.73 m² for young women and 130 ml/min/1.73 m² for men.[1] GFR also tends to be greater in bigger people so it is often corrected to a body surface area of 1.73 m². Strictly speaking however this correction should be for lean body mass and there is some controversy as to whether it should be performed in obese individuals.

What determines GFR?

The three physiological determinants of GFR are:
1. Ultrafiltration pressure (P_{UF})
2. Permeability of the glomerular capillary wall (k)
3. Surface area of capillary available for filtration (s)

$$GFR = P_{UF}.\ k.\ s$$

P_{UF} is determined by the hydrostatic pressure across the capillary wall (P) and the oncotic pressure of plasma proteins (π) which will oppose it.

$$P_{UF} = (P - \pi)$$

Furthermore, the pressure and protein gradients across the capillary wall will depend upon the difference between intracapillary and interstitial values.

Thus $P = (P_{GC} - P_{IF})$
$\pi = (\pi_{GC} - \pi_{IF})$

Where P_{GC} = glomerular capillary pressure
P_{IF} = pressure in the interstitial space
π_{GC} = glomerular capillary oncotic pressure
π_{IF} = oncotic pressure in the interstitial space.

Therefore GFR = k. s. $[(P_{GC} - P_{IF}) - (\pi_{GC} - \pi_{IF})]$

It is not possible to estimate these variables in humans except by using highly invasive methods such as renal biopsy, and mathematical modelling based upon assumptions of glomerular number and estimates of filtration surface area. GFR is therefore measured by testing the ability of the kidney to clear endogenous or exogenous substances.

Why is it important?

GFR is important because as it reduces, the ability to clear toxic waste products declines, leading to symptoms (nausea, fatigue, breathlessness), signs (hypertension, anaemia, fluid retention) and ultimately death, often from hyperkalaemia.

For reasons that are not completely clear but are multi-factorial, patients with chronic renal impairment are more prone to cardiovascular disease (CVD: ischaemic heart disease, stroke, peripheral vascular disease) and premature mortality. As there are readily available therapies to correct associated cardiovascular risks (such as statins, antihypertensives and anti-platelet drugs) the early identification and treatment of patients is perceived as a high clinical priority. Moreover an accelerated loss of GFR is a hallmark of established diabetic nephropathy so early detection of a reduced GFR is important.

How do you measure it?

In clinical practice, GFR is estimated from the clearance formula:

$$GFR = \frac{U.V}{P}$$

Where   U = urinary concentration of the clearance molecule
V = urine volume per unit time
P = plasma concentration ideally measured at the midpoint of the urine collection period

The ideal molecule to estimate GFR should be safe and non-toxic, be easy to measure, be freely filtered at the glomerular capillary and not have significant renal tubular absorption or excretion.

The gold standard substance is inulin (a polymer of fructose), but has drawbacks in the need for a steady-state intravenous infusion and accurately timed and complete urine collections. Other exogenous markers that have been used include radio-isotope labelled compounds such as ^{51}Cr EDTA or ^{125}I-iothalamate; or radiocontrast media such as iohexol. All are limited by expense, the need for injection, multiple blood samples and radiation concerns or iodine sensitivity.[1] They are therefore impractical for repeated use in routine clinical practice.

Creatinine is an endogenous product of muscle protein metabolism. In some ways it fulfils the criteria for an ideal marker to estimate GFR (eGFR). Its production is stable in the resting state, it is freely filtered at the glomerulus and is relatively cheap and easy to measure. However, it is secreted by the proximal tubule and this process can be affected by drugs such as cimetidine or trimethoprim. Extra renal excretion of creatinine in the gastro-intestinal tract increases with declining renal function. At low levels of GFR creatinine clearance tends to overestimate true values. Despite this, creatinine clearance is a reasonable estimate of GFR but of course depends upon a timed (usually 24 hour) urine collection.

In an attempt to avoid the need for urine collections, which are inconvenient for patients and need accurate timing with complete bladder emptying, serum (or plasma) creatinine alone has been used for many years as a proxy measure of GFR.

Serum levels, however, vary considerably with muscle bulk and can increase after vigorous exercise or a high meat protein meal. Moreover, the relationship of serum creatinine to GFR is non-linear so a reduction of 50% or more from normal would not be detected by a change in serum creatinine concentration (Figure 1).[2]

Figure 1: Relation of serum creatinine concentration to measured glomerular filtration rate (GFR)[2]

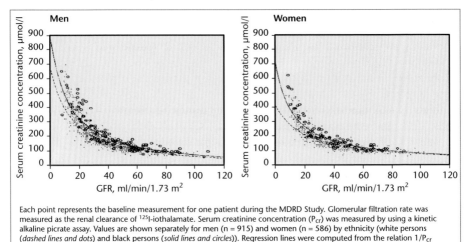

Each point represents the baseline measurement for one patient during the MDRD Study. Glomerular filtration rate was measured as the renal clearance of ^{125}I-iothalamate. Serum creatinine concentration (P_{cr}) was measured by using a kinetic alkaline picrate assay. Values are shown separately for men (n = 915) and women (n = 586) by ethnicity (white persons (*dashed lines and dots*) and black persons (*solid lines and circles*)). Regression lines were computed from the relation $1/P_{cr}$ compared with GFR. Black men (n = 113) have higher serum creatinine values than white men (n = 802) (p <0.001); black women (n = 84) have higher serum creatinine values than white women (n = 502) (p <0.001). To convert ml/min/1.73 m^2 to mL.s $^{-1}$.m $^{-2}$, multiply by 0.00963.

In patients with known chronic kidney disease (CKD) and an already increased serum creatinine, it is possible to get round some of these problems by plotting the inverse value against time, which creates a straight-line relationship.[3] This solution does not work for cross-sectional studies or for values much below 150 μmol/l.

Two mathematical methods to estimate GFR from serum creatinine are in common use. The Cockroft–Gault formula estimates creatinine clearance (CrCl) from the following:

$$CrCl \text{ (ml/min)} = 140 - age \text{ (years)} . \text{ body weight (kg)} . 1/SeCr . k$$

where   SeCr = serum creatinine
k = 1.23 for men and 1.05 for women

It can also be corrected for body surface by multiplying by 1.73/body surface area.

The drawbacks for Cockroft–Gault are the need for an accurate weight (and height if correcting for body surface area), the continuing problem of the bias introduced by obesity and fat mass and no correction for ethnicity. Moreover, it is an estimate of CrCl, not true GFR.[1]

The Modification of Diet in Renal Disease (MDRD) Study was set up to explore the effect of restriction of dietary protein intake on progression of renal disease. GFR was estimated using ^{125}I-iothalamate clearance and the majority of subjects had values <60 ml/min/1.73 m^2. Using values from 1,628 patients, formulae for the estimation of GFR already corrected for body surface area were derived. The simplest to use is the 4 point equation:

$$GFR \ (ml/min/1.73 \ m^2) = 175 \times SeCr \ (mg/dl)^{-1.154}. \ age \ (years)^{-0.203}$$
(convert mmol/l to mg/dl by dividing by 88.4)

Values are corrected by multiplying by 0.742 if female and 1.212 if black (Afro-Caribbean).[1,2]

Recently, in an attempt to improve accuracy a standardised method for SeCr has been developed by the Cleveland Clinic. Pathology laboratories can check their own methods against this standard and adjust their results accordingly. It is important to know if this correction is taking place before estimating GFR, as a correction factor may need to be applied. The quoted formula is for the standardised assay.[1]

Recently, plasma cystatin C has been proposed as a more accurate marker of GFR. It is freely filtered at the glomerulus but then reabsorbed and metabolised by the tubules. Thus its urine concentration is low and clearance cannot be estimated. At the moment it is uncertain if cystatin C measurement will prove to be an improvement over creatinine-based estimates of GFR.

Classification of CKD

In 2002 the US National Kidney Foundation proposed a classification of CKD based upon the MDRD equation (Table 1).[1,4] This has now been adopted by most national kidney disease specialist societies.[5]

Table 1: Stages of CKD as proposed by the US National Kidney Foundation[1]

Stage	eGFR (ml/min/1.73 m²)	Prevalence %	n (95% CI) millions (USA 2000)
1	>90 + kidney damage	2.8*	5.6 (4.0–7.2)
2	60–89 + kidney damage	2.8	5.7 (4.2–7.2)
3	30–59 ⎤	3.7	7.4 (6.0–8.9)
4	15–29 ⎥ For >3 months ± kidney damage	0.1	0.3 (0.02–0.5)
5	<15 ⎦	0.2	0.3**

*   Kidney damage defined as albuminuria and/or abnormal urinary sediment on more than 2 occasions over 3 months.
** Prevalence of stage 5 based upon US Renal Data Systems register of patients receiving renal replacement therapy and will not include those unrecognised with end-stage disease or who are too frail to tolerate dialysis.

All patients with an eGFR <60 ml/min/1.73 m² are said to have CKD irrespective of their urinalysis.

One of the drawbacks of this classification for patients with diabetes is that it does not map easily to the conventional classification of diabetic kidney disease (DKD) based upon albuminuria.[4] Moreover, both type 1 and type 2 diabetes patients may have an increased GFR in the early years of their disease and therapies (such as angiotensin-converting enzyme (ACE) inhibitors), which reduce albuminuria, may lead to a misclassification. A suggested correlation between CKD and DKD classes is shown in Table 2.

Table 2: Chronic kidney disease (CKD) and likelihood of diabetic kidney disease (DKD)

eGFR ml/min/1.73 m^2	CKD stage	Normoalbuminuria (AER <30 mg/day) (ACR < 2.5 mg/mmol men; <3.5 women)	Microalbuminuria (AER = 30–299 mg/day) ACR 2.5–30 mg/mmol men; 3.5–30 women)	Clinical nephropathy (AER >300 mg/day) (ACR > 30 mg/mmol)
>60	1 + 2	Normal*	Possible DKD**	DKD
30–59	3	Diabetes + CKD†	Probable DKD	DKD
<30	4 + 5	Diabetes + CKD†	DKD	DKD

*   Diabetic patients with normal albuminuria should be regarded as at risk of DKD.
** Microalbuminuria more likely to be due to DKD in type 1 than type 2 diabetes patients at normal GFR.
†   Therapies that reduce albuminuria such as ACE inhibitors may mask DKD.
    ACR: Albumin:creatinine ratio; AER: Albumin excretion rate.

At the moment many treatment guidelines for diabetes patients are based upon the detection of abnormal albuminuria usually by an albumin:creatinine ratio (ACR). The CKD classification does not replace or preclude routine measurement of ACR in patients with diabetes.[4]

How good is MDRD eGFR in diabetes patients?

There are now numerous studies comparing clearance derived measures of GFR with eGFR in diabetes.[6,7] As a general rule the MDRD equation underestimates true GFR significantly, particularly in patients with values >60 ml/min/1.73 m^2. Paradoxically, the Cockroft–Gault equation gives a closer estimate because it reports CrCl which tends to give higher values than the MDRD equation. Perhaps predictably, the equations are much better at identifying patients with GFR <60 ml/min/1.73 m^2. However a sensitivity of only 72% for a GFR less than this value has been reported in type 2 diabetes patients with increased albuminuria.[6]

It must be remembered that GFR varies considerably throughout the day depending upon exercise, food intake, hydration and in people with diabetes, prevailing glycaemia. Thus a single measure of GFR with a clearance method over a limited (usually 4 hour) period with the subject at rest may give a falsely high "snap shot" reading that might be corrected by a more stable serum creatinine derived estimate. Thus some caution needs to be exercised in interpreting straight comparisons of methods.

Notwithstanding the comparative accuracy of clearance derived versus eGFR in diabetes, the reported correlation between eGFR and mortality in the general population is reproduced in people with diabetes. In the South Tees Mortality Study, the adjusted hazard ratio (HR) for ischaemic heart disease was 3.6 and 8.1 fold higher for those with an eGFR of 30–59 and < 30 ml/min/1.73 m^2 respectively,[8] whilst for stroke the HRs were 1.9 and 5.9 respectively (Figure 2). These are higher than those reported for the total adult population in the USA.[9]

Figure 2: Kaplan–Meier estimates of death rates from the South Tees Mortality Study at 10 years. All-cause mortality by baseline estimated GFR (ml/min/1.73 m^2)[8]

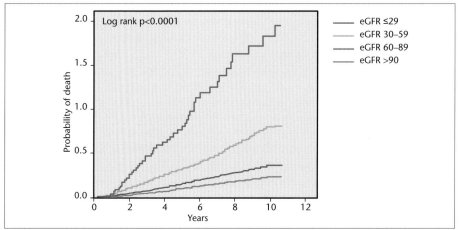

Thus regardless of the accuracy of eGFR it appears to be an important means of identifying patients with diabetes at high risk of CVD and a reduced value should prompt intensification of preventative strategies as well as a formal search for more specific renal complications such as anaemia and secondary hyperparathyroidism. It may also provide a more rational basis for clinical decision making, with regard to renally excreted drugs such as metformin, insulin and sulphonylureas.[10] One of the inconsistencies in this area is that the current definition of renal impairment in the British National Formulary does not map to the CKD staging in Table 1. For example, advice is given to avoid metformin in 'mild' renal impairment (GFR 20–50 ml/min), which equates to most of stage 3 and stages 4 & 5.[11] My own current practice is to review metformin use if eGFR <45 ml/min/1.73m^2. If kidney function is stable and metformin is strongly indicated then I continue with strict instructions to the patient to stop taking tablets if they become dehydrated for any reason, such as, coincident sickness and diarrhoea. A frequently asked question relates to the use of ACE inhibitors and/or angiotensin receptor-blocking drugs in the presence of renal impairment. The evidence is that these agents are effective in reducing progression of nephropathy in patients both with and without diabetes and stages 1–3 CKD. In more advanced renal impairment, an individual case-by-case decision must be made, but these patients should already be under specialist surveillance. A reduced eGFR should also form the basis for determining patient referral pathways for possible renal replacement therapy.[12] There is an urgent need for research to explore the utility of eGFR in these areas.

What should we do with the result?

A joint working party in the UK has published guidelines for general physicians and GPs.[5] Its recommendations for referral are summarised in a leaflet which is freely available from the Royal College of General Practitioners (RCGP) and are reproduced here (Table 3). Details can be found on the Renal Association website.[13] eGFR should be assessed at least annually in patients with stage 1 and 2 CKD and more frequently in stage 3, perhaps 3–6-monthly, depending on stability, but more frequently if changing therapy (such as intensifying antihypertensive treatment). Patients at stages 4 and 5 should be under regular specialist review. It has been pointed out that >30% of patients with type 2 diabetes may have an eGFR <60 ml/min/1.73 m^2 [14,15] and our own district register data for South Tees in 2004 confirms this figure. This is about six times that reported for the adult population in the UK, which of course includes those with diabetes. It is therefore important to refer only those stage 3 patients with difficult-to-control cardiovascular risk factors or who have a rapidly declining eGFR. Many elderly patients with a low GFR have stable values that do not necessarily need further investigation or specific treatment. It depends upon local arrangements whether referrals are made to a diabetes or renal service. For those patients with rapidly declining eGFR, then a direct renal referral is probably necessary. Many nephrologists have set up help lines for rapid advice without the need for referral of all in stage 3 CKD. For patients with more stable function but difficult to control risk factors, a diabetes referral may be more appropriate.

Conclusions

Although there are drawbacks in the use of eGFR for the monitoring of kidney function in diabetes, it remains a significant advance over SeCr alone. It serves as a method for identifying patients at high risk of CVD and should provide useful information on guiding therapy. The modified MDRD equation is currently recommended; however, it is not a precise measure of glomerular filtration and if this is required, then more accurate clearance methods should be used. Further research is needed on the utility of eGFR in clinical practice and less on the comparisons between methodologies.

Table 3: Criteria for referral of patients with CKD

Stages 1 + 2: eGFR >60 ml/min/1.73m^2 with signs of kidney disease (abnormal urinalysis) plus

- Malignant hypertension (urgent)
- Hyperkalaemia (K$^+$ >7 mmol/l) (urgent)
- Nephrotic syndrome (urgent)
- Isolated proteinuria (protein:creatinine ratio (PCR) >100 mg/mmol)
- Proteinuria and microscopic haematuria (PCR >100 mg/mmol)
- Diabetes with proteinuria (PCR >100 mg/mmol) but no retinopathy
- Macroscopic haematuria (after negative urological evaluation)
- Recurrent pulmonary oedema with normal left ventricular function
- Fall of eGFR of >15% during first 2 months on ACE inhibitors or angiotensin receptor blockers

Stage 3 – as above plus

- Progressive fall in GFR
- Microscopic haematuria (after negative urological tests if > 50 years old)
- Proteinuria (PCR >45 mg/mmol)
- Anaemia (after exclusion of other causes)
- Persistently abnormal serum potassium, calcium, phosphate (uncuffed sample)
- Suspected underlying systemic illness e.g. systemic lupus erythematosis, vasculitis, myeloma
- Uncontrolled hypertension (BP >150/90 mmHg on 3 agents)

Stages 4/5 (urgent)

All patients should be referred or at least discussed formally with a nephrologist.

References

1. Stevens LA, Coresh J, Greene T, Levey AS. Assessing kidney function – measured and estimated glomerular filtration rate. *N Engl J Med* 2006; **354:** 2473–83.

2. Levey AS, Bosch JP, Lewis JB et al. A more accurate method to estimate glomerular filtration rate from serum creatinine: a new prediction equation. Modification of Diet and Renal Disease Study Group. *Ann Intern Med* 1999; **130:** 461–70.

3. Jones RH, Hayakawa H, MacKay JD et al. Progression of diabetic nephropathy. *Lancet* 1979; **1:** 1105–6.

4. KDOQI™. KDOQI Clinical practice guidelines and clinical practice recommendations for diabetes and chronic kidney disease. *Am J Kidney Dis* 2007; **49** (2 suppl 2): S12–S154.

5. Joint Specialty Committee on Renal Medicine of the Royal College of Physicians and the Renal Association, and the Royal College of General Practitioners. *Chronic kidney disease in adults: UK guidelines for identification, management and referral.* London: Royal College of Physicians, 2006.

6. Rossing P, Rossing K, Gaede P et al. Monitoring kidney function in type 2 diabetic patients with incipient and overt diabetic nephropathy. *Diabetes Care* 2006; **29:** 1024–30.

7. Chudleigh RA, Dunseath G, Evans W et al. How reliable is estimation of glomerular filtration rate at diagnosis of type 2 diabetes? *Diabetes Care* 2007; **30:** 300–5.

8. Nag S, Bilous R, Kelly W et al. All cause and cardiovascular mortality in diabetic subjects increases significantly with reduced estimated glomerular filtration rate (eGFR): 10 years' data from the South Tees Diabetes Mortality Study. *Diabet Med* 2007; **24:** 10–7.

9. Go A, Chertow G, Fan D et al. Chronic kidney disease and the risks of death, cardiovascular events and hospitalisation. *N Engl J Med* 2004; **351:** 1296–305.

10. Anonymous. The patient, the drug and the kidney. *Drug Ther Bull* 2006; **44:** 89–95.

11. British National Formulary. Appendix 3. www.bnf.org Accessed June 2007.

12. New JP, O'Donoghue DJ, Middleton RJ et al. Time to move from serum creatinine to eGFR. *Diabet Med* 2006; **23:** 1047–9.

13. www.renal.org/CKDguide/ckd.html Accessed June 2007.

14. Middleton RJ, Foley RN, Hegarty J et al. The unrecognized prevalence of chronic kidney disease in diabetes. *Nephrol Dial Transplant* 2006; **21:** 88–92.

15. Bilo HJ, Logtenberg SJ, de Grauw WJ et al. Time to move from serum creatinine to eGFR (letter). *Diabet Med* 2007; **24:** 571.

New drug therapies for the treatment of diabetes

Professor Clifford J Bailey

Key points

- Several new therapies for the management of diabetes have recently become available in the UK, including new formulations of some established agents such as gliclazide and metformin, to alter bioavailability, extend activity and reduce side effects.
- Single tablet 'fixed-dose' combinations of a thiazolidinedione with metformin are available to reduce the pill burden of type 2 diabetes.
- The incretin mimetic exenatide is a subcutaneously injected stable analogue of the incretin hormone glucagon-like peptide-1 (GLP-1) that can be used as add-on therapy to metformin and/or a sulphonylurea to boost prandial insulin secretion without weight gain.
- Sitagliptin, an inhibitor of the enzyme dipeptidyl peptidase IV (DPP-4), prevents degradation of endogenous incretin hormones as another means of enhancing prandial insulin secretion.
- The cannabinoid receptor-1 (CB-1) inhibitor rimonabant suppresses appetite and promotes weight loss, and improves glycaemic control in patients with type 2 diabetes.
- Further incretin mimetics, DPP-4 inhibitors and CB-1 inhibitors are advanced in development.

Introduction

New therapies for the treatment of diabetes, particularly type 2 diabetes, are needed for several reasons: the prevalence of type 2 diabetes is increasing rapidly, the disease is highly heterogeneous and progressive; present pharmacological agents are often unable to sustain recommended glycaemic targets.

Diabetes in the UK

The diabetes epidemic continues to escalate, and recent figures for the UK suggest that about 3.6% of the population have been diagnosed with diabetes,[1] most of whom appear to have type 2 diabetes. A further three-quarters of a million people are believed to be undiagnosed in the UK and an additional 5% of the population is estimated to have impaired glucose tolerance.[2] Despite the efforts of healthcare professionals, less than half of patients with diabetes have a glycated haemoglobin (HbA_{1c}) $\leq 7.5\%$ and problably fewer than 25% have an $HbA_{1c} < 6.5\%$.

Addressing disease progression

The inevitably progressive nature of type 2 diabetes is associated with a continuous deterioration of pancreatic β-cell function in the presence of unremitting insulin resistance. Accordingly, anti-diabetic drug therapy requires periodic up-titration to match disease advancement, and combinations of differently acting anti-diabetic agents are often needed to treat the varying states of endocrine and metabolic dysregulation. Many type 2 diabetes patients eventually require insulin therapy, frequently accompanied by oral agents to counter insulin resistance or assist prandial insulin secretion. Thus, differently acting blood glucose-lowering agents are needed to manage different stages in the natural history of the type 2 diabetes disease process.[3] These agents should, as much as possible, offer benefits that will minimise the common cardiovascular and small vessel complications of diabetes. Ideally the choice of pharmacokinetic and pharmcodynamic properties will enable prescribers to circumvent the contra-indications and restrictions imposed by comorbidities and interactions with other medications.

New formulations and indications

Several established anti-diabetic agents have recently received new formulations or extended indications. A more bioavailable controlled-release formulation of gliclazide has been developed for once-daily administration, and a slow-release metformin formulation has been introduced to extend the duration of action and reduce gastro-intestinal (GI) side effects.[4,5] The European Medicines Evaluation Agency no longer contra-indicates use of a thiazolidinedione with insulin, and attitudes towards triple therapy with three differently acting oral agents or with insulin plus two oral agents appear to be more relaxed (provided all relevant contra-indications and monitoring are respected).

Single tablet combinations

Lower dosages of two differently acting blood glucose-lowering agents provide an opportunity for additive efficacy with fewer side effects.[6] To simplify combination therapy, several single tablet 'fixed-dose' combinations have been introduced (Table 1). The UK has received these therapies with greater caution than other parts of the world, despite more than one-third of type 2 diabetes patients already being treated with two or more different anti-diabetic medications. Given the large 'pill burden' of diabetes and the negative impact this can have on adherence, the use of single tablet combinations is likely to increase, and other combinations will be developed to incorporate emerging agents.

Table 1: Single tablet 'fixed-dose' combinations of oral anti-diabetic agents in the UK.

Trade name	Components	Strengths (mg)
Avandamet	Metformin + rosiglitazone	500:2, 1000:2, 1000:4
Competact*	Metformin + pioglitazone	850:15

* Competact is called Actoplusmet in some countries. Additional 'fixed-dose' combinations are approved in some countries outside the UK: these include Glucovance (metformin + glibenclamide), Metaglip (metformin + glipizide), Avaglim/Avandaryl (rosiglitazone + glimepiride), Tandemact/Duetact (pioglitazone + glimepiride). Janumet (sitagliptin + metformin) has been provisionally approved in the USA.

Incretin mimetics

March 2007 saw the UK launch of the first incretin mimetic 'exenatide'.[7] This is an analogue of the gut hormone glucagon-like peptide-1 (GLP-1). The background to this therapeutic approach is the physiological release of GLP-1 from the gut mucosa in response to a meal.[8,9] GLP-1 increases glucose-stimulated insulin secretion which enhances the prandial insulin response (so-called incretin effect) and reduces the glucose excursion. In addition, GLP-1 reduces glucagon secretion in a glucose-dependent manner, slows gastric emptying and exerts a satiety effect (Figure 1). Whether GLP-1 can preserve β-cell mass in human type 2 diabetes remains to be established.

Figure 1: Effects of the incretin hormones glucagon-like peptide-1 (GLP-1) and glucose-dependent insulinotropic peptide (GIP).

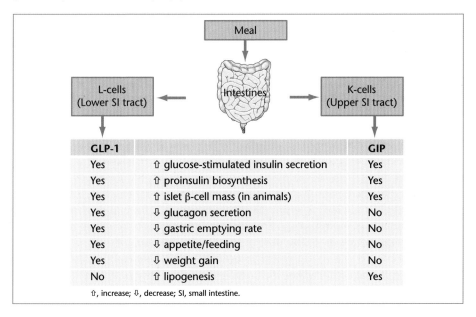

GLP-1		GIP
Yes	⇧ glucose-stimulated insulin secretion	Yes
Yes	⇧ proinsulin biosynthesis	Yes
Yes	⇧ islet β-cell mass (in animals)	Yes
Yes	⇩ glucagon secretion	No
Yes	⇩ gastric emptying rate	No
Yes	⇩ appetite/feeding	No
Yes	⇩ weight gain	No
No	⇧ lipogenesis	Yes

⇧, increase; ⇩, decrease; SI, small intestine.

The incretin effect is reduced in type 2 diabetes, and this is attributed, at least in part, to reduced secretion of GLP-1. The biological actions of GLP-1 remain essentially intact in type 2 diabetes, but administration of extra GLP-1 is not a practical therapeutic option because the peptide is degraded rapidly by the enzyme dipepidyl peptidase IV (DPP-4) which recognises and breaks the peptide at the N2 alanine residue (Figure 2). Exenatide is a GLP-1 analogue with a different N2 residue that confers resistance to degradation by DPP-4: exenatide retains the biological effects of GLP-1, enabling the incretin effect to be enhanced.

Figure 2: Amino acid sequences of human glucagon-like peptide-1 (GLP-1) 7-36 amide, and the GLP-1 analogue exenatide, showing the sequence homology.

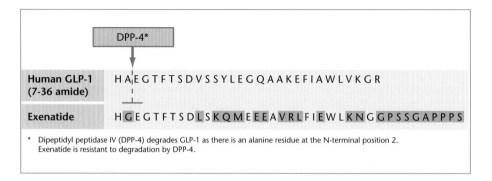

Exenatide, from the saliva of the Gila monster (*Heloderma suspectum*), a lizard native to the south western USA and northern Mexico, is a peptide, and is therefore administered by subcutaneous injection. Usually it is given twice daily during the hour before each of the morning and evening meals. Exenatide is available in pre-loaded pen injectors at either of two doses (5 μg and 10 μg) and is presently indicated for use as add-on therapy for type 2 diabetes patients inadequately contolled with metformin and/or a sulphonylurea.[7] In principle, exenatide should not cause clinical hypoglycaemia since its insulin-releasing and glucagon-suppressing effects do not occur at low blood-glucose concentrations. However, hypoglycaemia may occur when used with other blood glucose-lowering agents, especially sulphonylureas. Preferably begin with the 5 μg dose b.d. to minimise risk of hypoglycaemia and to reduce the prospect of nausea, which is a common early, but generally transient, effect presumed to result from delayed gastric emptying. The latter effect implies avoidance in patients with evidence of gastroparesis and reflux. Concurrent medications affected by gastric retention should be taken well before the exenatide injection, and drugs normally taken with food should, where possible, be taken with meals when exenatide is not used. Since exenatide is mostly eliminated by glomerular filtration, use in patients with severe renal disease (e.g. creatinine clearance <30 ml/min) is contra-indicated. Antibodies to exenatide have been detected in about one-third of patients treated, but anti-hyperglycaemic efficacy only appears to be reduced in about 3% of these patients.

A group of phase 3, randomised, double-blind, placebo-controlled trials examined the effect of add-on exenatide in patients inadequately controlled (mean HbA_{1c} 8.2–8.6%) with metformin and/or a sulphonylurea. The exenatide showed consistent dose-related glucose-lowering efficacy, achieving reductions in HbA_{1c} of 0.8–0.9% at the 10 μg dose over 6 months (Figure 3).[10] The 2-hour postprandial glucose concentration was reduced by about 4 mmol/l, and there was no increase in reported hypoglycaemic events with metformin, although hypoglycaemia was increased with a sulphonylurea. Body weight was reduced by 1.6–2.8 kg after 6 months of add-on exenatide, and further weight reductions occurred during the open-label trial extensions. This has been attributed mainly to a satiety effect of exenatide.

Figure 3: Effect of exenatide (5 µg b.d. or 10 µg b.d.) as add-on therapy to metformin in type 2 diabetes.[10]

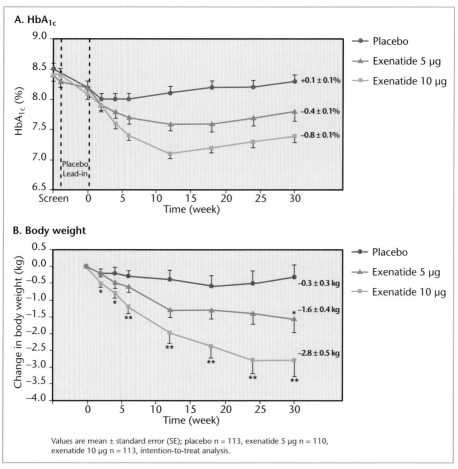

Values are mean ± standard error (SE); placebo n = 113, exenatide 5 µg n = 110, exenatide 10 µg n = 113, intention-to-treat analysis.

DPP-4 inhibitors

A related approach to anti-diabetic therapy is the inhibition of the DPP-4 enzyme to prevent the degradation of incretin hormones. This extends the half-lives of endogenous GLP-1 and certain other incretins such as glucose-dependent insulinotropic peptide (GIP), giving rise to an increased incretin response.[11] The first anti-diabetic agent in this new class of orally active DPP-4 inhibitors (termed gliptins) is 'sitagliptin', launched in the UK in April 2007.[12]

DPP-4 is a widespread dipeptidase enzyme that exists free in the circulation and tethered at the external surface of plasma membranes. It can cleave the N-terminal dipeptide from many of the peptides that have either an alanine or proline residue penultimate to the N-terminus (Figure 2). This disables or completely inactivates such peptides. Hence the inhibition of DPP-4 by a gliptin has the potential to extend the half-lives of many biologically active peptides, including hormones and other regulatory peptides that affect hunger–satiety balance, growth, vasoactivity, monocyte behaviour and GI motility as well as the incretin effect. While gliptins substantially raise the circulating concentrations of active GLP-1 and GIP, clinical studies to date have not identified any significant adverse effects. DPP-4 is also the CD-26 T-cell activating antigen, but inhibition of the dipeptidase activity has not been found to interfere with immune function as indicated by infections in the studies to date.

Sitagliptin is available in the UK as a 100 mg tablet to be taken once daily. It is highly selective for DPP-4 and almost totally inhibits DPP-4 activity for 24 hours, increasing active circulating concentrations of GLP-1 and GIP by 2–3 fold. This is associated with increased glucose-stimulated insulin secretion (relative to the prevailing level of glycaemia). The effect of GLP-1 to reduce glucagon secretion is also evident, although changes in satiety and gastric emptying have not been reported.

The indication for sitagliptin is add-on therapy for type 2 diabetes patients inadequately contolled with metformin or a thiazolidinedione.[12] This does not appear to cause clinical hypoglycaemia since (like exenatide and GLP-1) the insulin-releasing and glucagon-suppressing effects of sitagliptin do not occur at low blood-glucose concentrations. Absorption of sitagliptin is rapid (nearly 90% bioavailability in 1–4 hours) and unaffected by food. About one-third is protein bound and almost 80% is eliminated unchanged in the urine. More is probably eliminated by renal tubular secretion via the organic anion transporter-3 than by glomerular filtration. Nevertheless sitagliptin is not recommended if creatinine clearance is <50 ml/min. About 16% of sitagliptin is metabolised, mainly by the P450 isoenzymes CYP3A4 and CYP2C8, giving rise to several inactive metabolites. Sitagliptin does not appear to induce or inhibit P450 isoenzymes and no significant drug interactions have been identified other than a small increase in digoxin concentrations.

During phase 3 randomised, double-blind, placebo-controlled trials, sitagliptin add-on therapy was assessed in type 2 diabetes patients inadequately controlled (mean HbA_{1c} 8.0–8.1%) with metformin or pioglitazone for 24 weeks (Figure 4). Addition of sitagliptin (100 mg o.d.) reduced mean HbA_{1c} by about 0.7%, and did not alter body-weight or the incidence of hypoglycaemia compared with addition of placebo. As add-on to metformin, sitagliptin reduced the 2-hour postprandial glucose concentration by about 3 mmol/l.[13]

Figure 4: Effect of sitagliptin (100 mg o.d.) as add-on therapy to metformin in type 2 diabetes.[13]

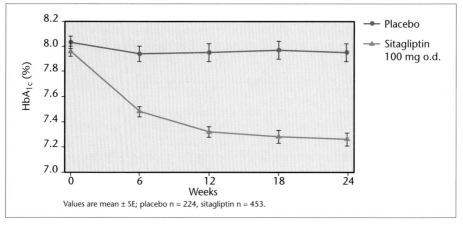

Values are mean ± SE; placebo n = 224, sitagliptin n = 453.

Cannabinoid receptor-1 inhibitors

Although a role of anti-obesity agents in the management of type 2 diabetes is not universally accepted, it is well recognised that weight loss amongst overweight and obese patients improves metabolic control. Overactivity of the endocannabinoid system has been observed in many conditions of excess adiposity.[14] This involves increased production of endogenous cannabinoids such as 2-arachidonoylglycerol (2-AG) and anandamide as well as increased expression of cannabinoid receptors, especially type 1 (CB-1). The CB-1 receptors are abundant in regions of the hypothalamus where they mediate the stimulation of appetite, and in visceral fat where they promote lipogenesis. Selective blockade of CB-1 receptors curbs excess appetite and adipose deposition, facilitating weight loss and improved metabolic control. Recently, this approach has been shown to benefit weight management and glycaemic control in overweight and obese type 2 diabetes patients.

The first CB-1 receptor blocker, rimonabant, was launched in the UK in July 2006. It is indicated for use as an adjunct to diet and exercise for the treatment of obesity [body mass index (BMI) ≥30 kg/m²], or overweight (BMI ≥27 kg/m²) with one or more associated risk factors such as type 2 diabetes or dyslipidaemia.[15] In a series of randomised, double-blind, placebo-controlled trials in non-diabetic subjects, following a dietary intake that was reduced by 600 kcal/day, addition of rimonabant 20 mg o.d. for 1 year reduced body weight by about 5 kg and waist circumference by >4 cm more than placebo.[16]

A recent double-blind placebo-controlled study in overweight and obese type 2 diabetes patients inadequately controlled (mean HbA_{1c} about 7.3%) with metformin or a sulphonylurea noted that a reduction of 600 kcal/day with randomisation to add-on rimonabant (20 mg o.d.) for 1 year resulted in about 4 kg more weight loss than the reduced diet with add-on placebo (Figure 5). Rimonabant was also associated with a 0.6% reduction in HbA_{1c} compared with a 0.1% gain in the placebo group.[17] The decrease in HbA_{1c} would appear to be greater than expected for the weight loss alone, raising the possibility of additional anti-hyperglycaemic benefits of rimonabant. Small increases in high density lipoprotein and decreases in triglyceride were noted with rimonabant.

Figure 5: Effect of rimonabant (5 mg and 20 mg o.d.) as add-on therapy to metformin or a sulphonylurea in type 2 diabetes.[17]

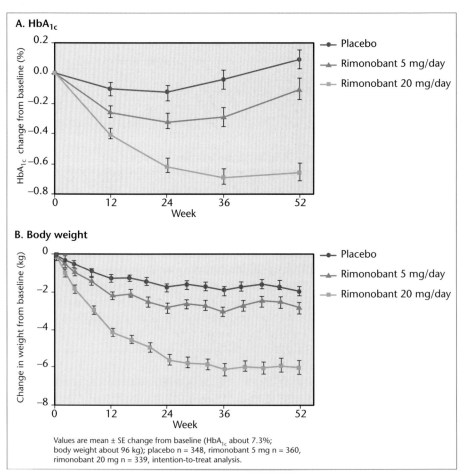

Values are mean ± SE change from baseline (HbA_{1c} about 7.3%; body weight about 96 kg); placebo n = 348, rimonabant 5 mg n = 360, rimonabant 20 mg n = 339, intention-to-treat analysis.

A 0.5% greater reduction in HbA_{1c} and a 4 kg greater reduction in body weight than placebo has been reported with rimonabant (20 mg o.d. for 6 months) in overweight and obese type 2 diabetes patients, inadequately controlled (mean HbA_{1c} 7.9%) by diet/ exercise alone.

Since rimonabant has been associated with an increased occurrence of depressive disorders, anxiety and dizziness, patients with serious psychiatric illness are contra-indicated.[15] Substantial hepatic metabolism of rimonabant by CYP3A4 implies that caution should be taken with drugs that induce, inhibit or are metabolised by this P450 isoenzyme. Severe liver or renal diseases are also exclusions.

Future anti-diabetic therapies

In various countries outside of the UK there are additional anti-diabetic therapies available, such as the soluble amylin analogue 'pramlintide', which is injected pre-meals as an adjunct to insulin therapy in type 1 or type 2 diabetes patients. Pramlintide reduces glucagon, slows gastric emptying and exerts a satiety effect, enabling glycaemic control to be improved, usually with a reduction of insulin dose and a decrease in weight.[18]

Several further incretin mimetic therapies are advanced in development. These include liraglutide, which is a long-acting (once-daily) GLP-1 formulation in which GLP-1 is linked to a fatty acid that enables it to bind to albumin and prolong its survival in the circulation. Longer acting, possibly once-weekly or once-monthly, injections of GLP-1 analogues are also under investigation. Additional DPP-4 inhibitors are nearing completion of registration studies: these include vildagliptin and saxagliptin. New CB-1 inhibitors are proceeding quickly in development, but these are at earlier stages in the clinical trials process.

Many interesting possibilities for the future treatment of diabetes have received preclinical and early clinical investigation.[19,20] For example, inhibitors of the renal glucose transporter SGLT2 provide a mechanism to eliminate excess glucose in the urine, while glucokinase activators can enhance glucose-induced insulin secretion and increase hepatic glucose uptake and metabolism. Proof of principle for non-peptide insulin mimetics and potentiators has also been obtained. Although recently developed peroxisome proliferator-activated receptor-alpha/gamma (dual PPARα/γ) agonists have not proceeded into clinical use due to side effects, selective PPAR agonists are proceeding in early development.

Conclusion

This is a crucial time for anti-diabetic therapy: the importance of achieving and maintaining glycaemic targets whenever possible and practicable is established. For type 2 diabetes patients the progressive nature of the disease is appreciated, and the likely need to address different aspects of disease pathophysiology with different agents and combination therapies is accepted. Several new therapies have become available to assist in these missions.

References

1. Kenny C. Diabetes and the quality and outcomes framework. *BMJ* 2005; **331**: 1097–8.

2. International Diabetes Federation. *Diabetes Atlas.* (Third edn). Brussels: International Diabetes Federation, 2006; 64–5.

3. Krentz AJ, Bailey CJ. Oral antidiabetic agents. Current role in type 2 diabetes mellitus. *Drugs* 2005; **65**: 385–411.

4. Servier Laboratories Limited. *Diamicron 30 mg MR. Summary of Product Characteristics.* February 2007.

5. Merck Pharmaceuticals *Glucophage SR 500 mg prolonged release tablets. Summary of Product Characteristics.* May 2006.

6. Bailey CJ. Whence and whither the fixed-dose combination? *Diab Vasc Dis Res* 2005; **2**: 51–3.

7. Eli Lilly and Company Limited. *Byetta 5 micrograms solution for injection, prefilled pen. Byetta 10 micrograms solution for injection, prefilled pen. Summary of Product Characteristics.* December 2006.

8. Holst JJ. Glucagon-like peptide-1: from extract to agent. The Claude Bernard Lecture, 2005. *Diabetologia* 2006; **49**: 253–60.

9. Drucker DJ. The role of gut hormones in glucose homeostasis. *J Clin Invest* 2007; **117**: 24–32.

10. DeFronzo RA, Ratner RE, Han J *et al.* Effects of exenatide (exendin-4) on glycemic control and weight over 30 weeks in metformin-treated patients with type 2 diabetes. *Diabetes Care* 2005; **28**: 1092–100.

11. Green BD, Flatt PR, Bailey CJ. Dipeptidyl peptidase IV (DPP IV) inhibitors: a newly emerging drug class for the treatment of type 2 diabetes. *Diab Vasc Dis Res* 2006; **3**: 159–65.

12. Merck Sharp & Dohme Limited. *Januvia 100 mg film-coated tablets. Summary of Product Characteristics.* April 2007.

13. Charbonnel B, Karasik A, Liu J *et al.* Efficacy and safety of the dipeptidyl peptidase-4 inhibitor sitagliptin added to ongoing metformin therapy in patients with type 2 diabetes inadequately controlled with metformin alone. *Diabetes Care* 2006; **29**: 2638–43.

14. Matias I, Gonthier MP, Orlando P *et al.* Regulation, function and dysregulation of endocannabinoids in models of adipose and beta-pancreatic cells and in obesity and hyperglycemia. *J Clin Endocrinol Metab* 2006; **91**: 3171–80.

15. Sanofi-Aventis. *Acomplia 20 mg film-coated tablets. Summary of Product Characteristics.* June 2006.

16. Van Gaal LF, Rissanen AM, Scheen AJ *et al.* Effects of the cannabinoid-1 receptor blocker rimonabant on weight reduction and cardiovascular risk factors in overweight patients: 1-year experience from the RIO-Europe study. *Lancet* 2005; **365**: 1389–97.

17. Scheen AJ, Finer N, Hollander P *et al.* Efficacy and tolerability of rimonabant in overweight or obese patients with type 2 diabetes: a randomised controlled study. *Lancet* 2006; **368**: 1660–72.

18. Day C. New therapies available for the treatment of type 2 diabetes. *Europ Diab Nursing* 2006; **3**: 65–70.

19. Bailey CJ. New drugs for the treatment of diabetes mellitus. In: DeFronzo RA, Ferrannini E, Keen H, Zimmet P (Eds). *International Textbook of Diabetes Mellitus.* (Third edn). Chichester: John Wiley, 2004.

20. Bailey CJ. Treating insulin resistance: future prospects. *Diab Vasc Dis Res* 2007; **4**: 20–31.

Implications of recent clinical trials of thiazolidinediones in type 2 diabetes

Dr Marc Evans, Dr Lucy Holder, Dr Raj Peter

Key points

- At lower glycosylated haemoglobin (HbA_{1c}) levels (7–7.5%), postprandial glucose (PPG) rather than fasting glucose appears to be more important. Hence, assessing fasting as well as PPG levels may aid in a tailored therapeutic approach to achieve optimal glycaemic control.
- The durability of glycaemic control appears to be a major benefit of thiazolidinedione (TZD) therapy.
- TZD therapy is associated with oedema, weight gain and heart failure risk. In addition, while the overall cardiovascular (CV) safety of rosiglitazone is unclear, data from the RECORD interim analysis appear reassuring. The results of specifically designed studies evaluating the CV effects of the TZDs are awaited to further address this issue.
- Pioglitazone appeared to be associated with a CV outcome benefit in high-risk patients. The apparent CV differences between rosiglitazone and pioglitazone cannot be completely accounted for on the basis of differing metabolic effects, raising the question of the potential for a threshold baseline CV risk effect for the benefits of TZDs on outcome.
- The overall risk–benefit profile of TZD therapy needs close evaluation on an individual patient basis.

Introduction

Insulin resistance and β-cell dysfunction are core features in the pathohysiology of type 2 diabetes, resulting in progressive elevations in fasting and postprandial blood glucose levels. The precise natural history of these glycaemic excursions is unclear and an understanding of these issues may have profound therapeutic implications.

The thiazolidinediones (TZDs) are blood glucose-lowering agents and are agonists for the nuclear hormone receptor peroxisome proliferator-activated receptor γ, which modulates gene expression resulting in increased insulin sensitivity in muscle, liver and adipose tissue, and may have the potential to produce more sustained glucose control.

The effect of any oral hypoglycaemic therapy on cardiovascular (CV) outcomes is particularly important, since more than 65% of deaths in patients with type 2 diabetes are from CV causes. Over the last year, three major clinical trials conducted in 14,957 patients have reported evaluating the effects of the TZDs on CV outcomes, disease progression and microvascular disease. The observations of these studies may have significant implications and have provided further insight into the long-term safety profile of these agents.

Postprandial blood glucose and type 2 diabetes

The predominant focus of glucose-lowering therapy has been on glycosylated haemoglobin (HbA$_{1c}$), with a strong emphasis on fasting plasma glucose (FPG). This has been partly due to the fact that the exact relationship between the various glycaemic indices has been poorly understood. Monnier and colleagues previously demonstrated the relationship between these variables is dependant on overall glycaemic status, with the contribution of PPG being predominant in the relatively well controlled (HbA$_{1c}$<7.3%), while the contribution of fasting glucose increases as glycaemia deteriorates.[1]

The years preceding the development of type 2 diabetes are characterised by a progressive decline in both insulin sensitivity and first-phase insulin secretion.[2] Postprandial hyperglycaemia may thus precede fasting hyperglycaemia.[1]

Using continuous glucose monitoring, 130 subjects with type 2 diabetes were stratified into five groups of HbA$_{1c}$ (<6.5%, 6.5–6.9%, 7.0–7.9%, 8.0–8.9% and ≥9.0%) and daytime glucose profiles plotted.[3] The daytime glucose profiles were analysed with respect to three study periods: daytime postprandial period (3–4 hours after meals); nocturnal fasting period (midnight to prebreakfast period) and morning period (1 hour before breakfast and ending 3 hours later). This unusual morning period was chosen by the authors to account for the 'dawn' and 'extended dawn' phenomenon.[4]

The first significant change in mean glucose levels was for daytime PPG with progressive changes seen from groups 1 to 5. The first significant difference was observed between group 1 (HbA$_{1c}$<6.5%) and group 2 (HbA$_{1c}$ between 6.5% and 6.9%); [6.4 mmol/l, 95% confidence interval (CI): 6.1–6.7 vs. 7.7 mmol/l; 95% CI: 7.0–8.4; p = 0.0004]. These differences were followed by changes in mean glucose concentrations for the morning period. Mean glucose concentrations increased with worsening HbA$_{1c}$ from groups 2 to 5; with the first statistically significant difference occurring between group 2 and group 3 (7.5 mmol/l; 95% CI: 6.8–8.3 vs. 9.3 mmol/l; 95% CI: 8.7–10.0; p = 0.0003). However, no statistically significant differences were observed between groups 1 and 2. For nocturnal fasting periods the first difference was noted between group 3 and 4 (6.3 mmol/l; 95% CI: 5.7–6.9 vs. 8.4 mmol/l; 95% CI: 7.7–9.3; p<0.0001) with a further deterioration in group 5.

A progressive loss in post-meal glycaemic control precedes a stepwise deterioration in fasting glucose as part of the natural history of type 2 diabetes. This study may also provide an explanation for patients who fail to achieve HbA$_{1c}$<7% but have near-normal FPG concentrations. The failure in optimising glycaemic control in this context may be related to persistent elevation of PPG.

The effects of TZD therapy on glycaemic control in people with type 2 diabetes

The ADOPT study evaluated rosiglitazone, metformin and glibenclamide as monotherapy for 4,360 recently diagnosed (<3 years) patients with type 2 diabetes over a median of 4 years, with the primary outcome being time to monotherapy failure defined as sustained FPG >10 mmol/l on maximal dose.[5] On study entry, subjects were randomised to receive 2.5 mg daily of glibenclamide, 500 mg daily of metformin or 4 mg daily of rosiglitazone with subsequent dose escalations occurring when fasting glucose levels increased beyond 7.8 mmol/l. Once patients reached the primary endpoint, they were excluded from further analysis, thus data for the pre-specified secondary endpoints including HbA_{1c}, insulin sensitivity and β-cell function were only obtained from those with FPG levels sustained at <10 mmol/l.

The cumulative incidence of monotherapy failure at 5 years was 15% for rosiglitazone, 21% for metformin and 34% for glibenclamide, representing a risk reduction of 32% for rosiglitazone as compared with metformin and 63% as compared with glibenclamide (p<0.001) (Figure 1).

Figure 1: Kaplan–Meier estimates of the cumulative incidence of monotherapy failure (FPG >10mmol/l) at 5 years from ADOPT.[5]

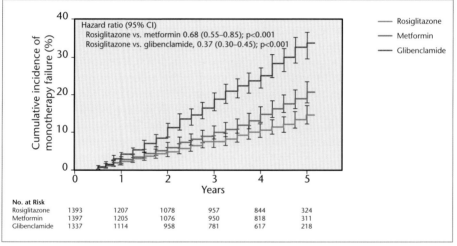

β-cell function improved more in the glibenclamide group during the first 6 months (mean ratio of 6-month value to baseline: 1.45), than in the rosiglitazone group (1.17) or metformin group (1.16). Thereafter, β-cell function declined in all groups; the annual rate of decline after 6 months was greatest in the glibenclamide group (6.1%), intermediate in the metformin group (3.1%) and least in the rosiglitazone group (2.0%). The rates of β-cell function decline were significantly greater in the glibenclamide (p<0.001) and metformin groups (p = 0.02) compared with rosiglitazone. In addition, after 5 years, HbA_{1c} was significantly lower with rosiglitazone compared with both metformin (0.13%, p = 0.002) and glibenclamide (0.42%, p<0.001) (Figure 2).

Figure 2: Time–course analysis: HbA$_{1c}$ over time, according to treatment group.[5]

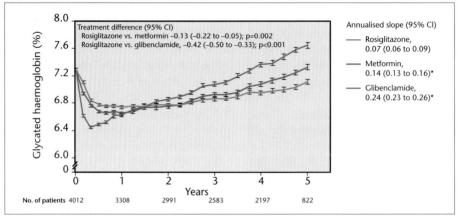

This study was not powered or designed to evaluate CV events. The proportion of patients experiencing heart failure (HF) in the rosiglitazone group was 1.5% compared with 1.3% (p = 0.52) of patients receiving metformin and 0.6% (p = 0.05) receiving glibenclamide. The incidence of HF was in line with that reported in previous trials and as indicated in the rosiglitazone Summary of Product Characteristics. Rosiglitazone was associated with more weight gain and oedema than metformin or glibenclamide but with fewer gastrointestinal events than metformin and less hypoglycaemia than glibenclamide. A higher rate of fractures was an unexpected observation in the rosiglitazone group. This was confined to the female population and involved an increased incidence of fractures involving the humerus, hand and foot. There was, however, no increase in the incidence of hip fractures and the mechanisms and clinical implications of these observations are unclear.

This study demonstrated that rosiglitazone was associated with the greatest durability of glycaemic control as defined by FPG <10 mmol/l. Patients were recruited into the trial over a 1-year period, with the last measurement taken at 5 years. Thus, measurements taken at the end of 5 years do not accurately represent the results of 5 years of treatment in the full-study population. At years 2, 3 and 4 following randomisation, 78%, 69% and 60% of subjects receiving rosiglitazone maintained FPG <10 mmol/l as compared with 71%, 58% and 46% in the glibenclamide group, implying that monotherapy is insufficient to maintain suitable glycaemic control in a significant proportion of patients.

The CV implications of TZD therapy

The majority of rosiglitazone data to date has focused on glucose control. Nissen and Wolski conducted a meta-analysis of trials comparing rosiglitazone with placebo or active comparators to assess its effects on CV outcomes.[6]

Only 42 of 116 screened trials met the inclusion criteria for meta-analysis. Of those initially assessed, 48 trials had an active comparator group, a similar duration of treatment and more than 24 weeks of drug exposure, however six of these did not report CV events. In the remaining trials, 15,565 patients were randomised to receive rosiglitazone and 12,282 to non-rosiglitazone comparators. Data from this meta-analysis were combined by means of a fixed-effects model; the mean age of subjects was approximately 56 years, with a mean baseline HbA_{1c} of 8.2%. In the rosiglitazone group, as compared with the control group, the odds ratio for myocardial infarction (MI) was 1.43 (95% CI 1.03–1.98, p = 0.03) and the odds ratio for death from CV causes was 1.64 (95% CI 0.98–2.74, p = 0.06) reflecting a 1 in 250 myocardial event rate per 2.2 years of therapy with rosiglitazone. These data outwardly suggest that, as compared with placebo or other oral hypoglycaemic agents, rosiglitazone was associated with a significant increase in the risk of MI and a non-significant increase in the risk of death from vascular disease, with a possible mechanism involving the effects of an increase in intravascular volume on myocardial oxygen demands. These observations are however based on limited trial data (42 out of 116) with many contributing studies being small scale and short term primarily designed to evaluate glycaemic control. In addition, they had no event adjudication and an imbalance in follow-up, with more patients in the control group withdrawing due to hyperglycaemia. Furthermore, trials with no MIs were excluded and overall rates of adverse events are low. The actual numbers of adverse events are relatively small (MI: 86 vs. 72; CV death: 39 vs. 22), thus, even small changes in the classification of these events could lead to significantly different odds ratios. Furthermore, analysis of the largest individual rosiglitazone active comparator trial (ADOPT) demonstrates similar rates of adverse CV events for rosiglitazone, metformin and glibenclamide monotherapy (Table 1).[7] A more accurate evaluation of the CV effects of rosiglitazone would be derived from patient source data or specifically-designed studies to evaluate CV events, such as the ongoing Rosiglitazone Evaluated for Cardiovascular and Regulation of Glycaemia in Diabetes (RECORD) trial.

Table 1: Major adverse CV events in the ADOPT study.[7]

	Rosiglitazone (n=1456)	Metformin (n=1454)	Glibenclamide (n=1441)
MACE			
Events	40	37	30
Hazard ratio (95% CI)	–	1.11 (0.71–1.74)	1.19 (0.74–1.91)
All cardiovascular deaths			
Events	5	4	8
Hazard ratio (95% CI)	–	1.30 (0.35–4.86)	0.58 (0.19–1.78)
Myocardial infarction serious adverse events			
Events	24	20	14
Hazard ratio (95% CI)	–	1.23 (0.68–2.22)	1.52 (0.79–2.94)
Myocardial ischaemia adverse events			
Events	106	111	82
Hazard ratio (95% CI)	–	0.99 (0.76–1.30)	1.18 (0.88–1.57)

MACE: Major adverse cardiovascular event [all CV deaths, MI serious adverse events (fatal and non-fatal), and stroke serious adverse events (fatal and non-fatal)].

Rosiglitazone evaluated for CV outcomes – an interim analysis

The RECORD trial is a long-term, multicentre, randomised, open-label study comparing CV outcomes in patients with type 2 diabetes treated with rosiglitazone plus metformin or sulphonylurea with outcomes in patients treated with metformin plus sulphonylurea. Following the recent meta-analysis of the CV safety of rosiglitazone, an interim report from this study was presented.[8]

A total of 4,447 patients (baseline HbA_{1c} 7.9%) receiving metformin or sulphonylurea monotherapy were randomly assigned to receive add-on rosiglitazone (2,220) or a combination of metformin plus sulphonylurea (2,227). If the HbA_{1c} exceeded 7.0% after 8 weeks of treatment, the doses of study drugs were increased to maximum (8 mg rosiglitazone, 2,550 mg metformin, 15 mg glibenclamide, 240 mg gliclazide and 4 mg glimepiride). If HbA_{1c} exceeded 8.5%, a third agent was added in the rosiglitazone group, while insulin was initiated for patients in the control group. If patients in the rosiglitazone group receiving triple therapy had HbA_{1c} levels >8.5% then rosiglitazone was discontinued and insulin commenced. The primary endpoint was hospitalisation or death from CV causes, with a mean follow up of 3.75 years. A total of 217 patients in the rosiglitazone group and 202 in the control group had the adjudicated primary endpoint (hazard ratio 1.08; 95% CI 0.89–1.31), with no statistically significant difference between the rosiglitazone and control groups regarding death from CV causes and MI (Figures 3&4).

Figure 3: Time–course analysis: primary endpoint (adjudicated) first occurrence of CV death or hospitalisation.[8]

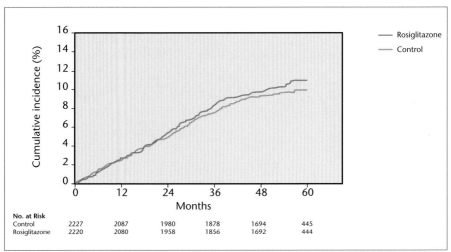

Figure 4: Time–course analysis: time to first occurrence of acute MI.[8]

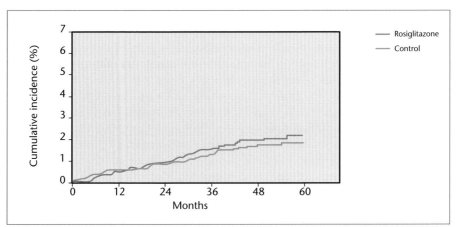

Approximately 10% of patients were lost to follow-up, while the annual event rate was low (3.15% per year), reflecting the impact of concomitant cardioprotective therapies or potential difficulties with event ascertainment. Patients in the rosiglitazone group had a higher risk of congestive HF (32 versus 17 adjudicated events). 6.5% of patients in the rosiglitazone group required insulin as opposed to 10.9% in the control group, with 1,626 patients in the rosiglitazone group and 1,476 in the control group still receiving their allocated therapy at 3.75 years. This study has several strengths in that it was a large, randomised, long-term study designed to assess the CV safety of rosiglitazone in the context of dual agent combination therapy, with all reported CV endpoints undergoing independent adjudication. It is however, non-blinded, with a low event rate and significant drop out rate and is designed as a non-inferiority study, all of which may limit the statistical power of the study to detect differences.

Pioglitazone and CV deaths

The PROactive study, a 3-year, double-blind, randomised, parallel-group, secondary-prevention study (approximately half of the patients had suffered a previous MI, a third had undergone coronary artery revascularisation, a fifth had presented with symptomatic arterial disease and a fifth had suffered a stroke), was designed to investigate whether the addition of pioglitazone to best-practice could reduce the incidence of further macrovascular events in 5,238 patients with type 2 diabetes.[9] Patients were randomised to receive pioglitazone or placebo, for a mean duration for 34.5 months, with investigators encouraged to optimise glycaemic therapy to a target $HbA_{1c}<6.5\%$. The primary endpoint was a composite of all-cause mortality, non-fatal MI, stroke, acute coronary syndrome, endovascular or surgical intervention on the coronary or leg arteries and major leg amputation. The secondary endpoint was a composite of all-cause mortality, non-fatal MI and stroke.

Pioglitazone was associated with a non-significant 10% relative risk reduction in the primary endpoint (p = 0.095), compared with placebo. Coronary heart disease events, stroke and CV deaths were lower in the pioglitazone group, however lower limb revascularisations were higher in the pioglitazone group resulting in the primary composite end-point being missed. Significantly more patients receiving placebo (n = 358) experienced the principal secondary endpoint than patients receiving pioglitazone (n = 301, p = 0.027), equating to a significant 16% relative risk reduction with pioglitazone (p = 0.027) (Figure 5).

Adding pioglitazone to best practice significantly improved glycaemic control (HbA_{1c} absolute change from baseline: -0.8% vs. -0.3%; p <0.0001) and reduced dyslipidaemia [percentage change in low-density lipoprotein (LDL)/high-density lipoprotein (HDL) ratio: -9.5 vs. -4.2; p<0.0001; change in triglycerides: -11.4% vs. -1.8%; p<0.0001]. The glycaemic benefits of pioglitazone may have been partly the consequence of sub-optimal therapeutic escalation in the placebo group.

Pioglitazone was also associated with a reduced systolic blood pressure (median change: -3 vs. 0 mmHg; p = 0.03) and reduced progression to insulin (53%; p<0.001). In this study, the median duration of type 2 diabetes was 9 years, despite which, pioglitazone showed an insulin-sparing effect manifested as either reducing the requirement to initiate insulin or reducing the dose of insulin in patients already receiving it.

Figure 5: Time to principal secondary endpoint in the PROactive study.[9]

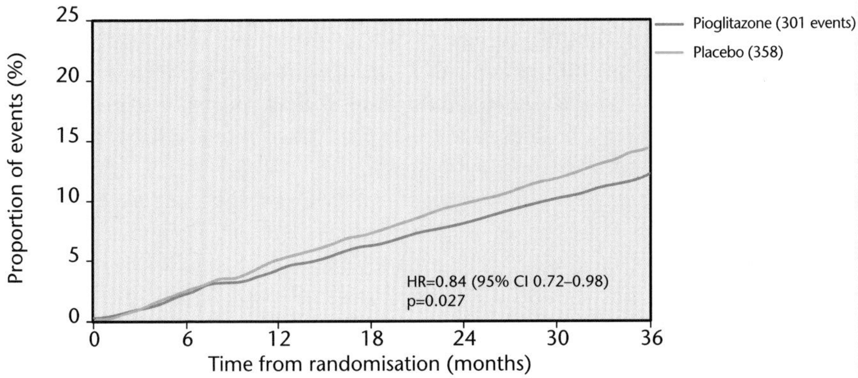

No. at Risk						
Pioglitazone	2536	2487	2435	2381	2336	396
Placebo	2566	2504	2442	2371	2315	390

HR, hazard ratio; CI, confidence interval

Kaplan–Meier estimates indicated that pioglitazone prevented 21 MIs, strokes or deaths for every 1000 patients treated over a 3-year period (one major CV event avoided for every 48 patients treated). In patients with a history of MI, pioglitazone reduced the risk of recurrent MI by 28% (p = 0.045),[10] while in patients with a prior history of stroke, pioglitazone reduced the risk of recurrent stroke by 47% (p = 0.0085).[11]

Although pioglitazone increased the incidence of reported HF, *post-hoc* independent adjudication confirmed that there was no inter-group difference in HF-related mortality (0.6% of patients from each group).[12] The review also confirmed the accuracy of the original investigator diagnoses of serious HF.[12] Despite this higher incidence of reported HF with pioglitazone, the risk of subsequent death or CV events was similar compared with placebo. Consequently, the overall benefit of reduction in macrovascular events with pioglitazone was not offset by worsened HF sequelae in these high-risk patients. Adverse events seen in PROactive were similar to those seen in both ADOPT and the RECORD interim analysis, with an almost doubling in the incidence of oedema in the absence of HF (21.6% vs. 13%) and an increase in weight of 3.6 kg, with weight gain leading to study cessation occurring in 0.8% of the pioglitazone group as compared with 0.2% in the control group. A higher incidence of pneumonia (2.1% vs. 1.3%) was also reported in the pioglitazone group.

In the setting of optimised multiple risk factor management, with intensive lipid and blood pressure reduction along with combination anti-platelet therapy, the absolute clinical and cost-effectiveness of the observations from PROactive are unclear.

Conclusion

In patients with a $HbA_{1c} > 8\%$, fasting hyperglycaemia appears to be the most pertinent therapeutic target. Once these glycaemic parameters have been appropriately addressed, and if HbA_{1c} remains sub-optimal (>7%), then both quantifying and treating PPG levels would be a logical therapeutic step. Such a concept has implications for blood glucose monitoring strategies and may lead to an increased use of agents that specifically target postprandial hyperglycaemia.

Glycaemic control appears to be a benefit of TZD therapy; the risk–benefit profile of these therapies is however an important consideration. Both rosiglitazone and pioglitazone are associated with weight gain, oedema, HF, and an increased risk of fractures in women. The overall CV safety profile of rosiglitazone is unclear, while PROactive suggested a CV benefit with pioglitazone. The current CV data for both TZDs is based on patient populations of markedly different risk, raising the question as to whether there is a threshold of risk that may impact on the outcome benefits of TZD therapy. It is, however, currently impossible to assess the 'class' effect on CV disease and the results of several large ongoing studies are awaited to address this issue.

References

1. Monnier L, Lapinski H, Colette C. Contributions of fasting and postprandial plasma glucose increments to the overall diurnal hyperglycaemia of type 2 diabetic patients: variations with increasing levels of HbA_{1c}. *Diabetes Care* 2003; **26**: 881–5.

2. Weyer C, Bogardus C, Mott DM, Pratley RE. The natural history of insulin secretory dysfunction and insulin resistance in the pathogenesis of type 2 diabetes mellitus. *J Clin Invest* 1999; **104**: 787–94.

3. Monnier L, Colette C, Dunseath G, Owens D. The loss of postprandial glycaemic control precedes stepwise deterioration of fasting with worsening diabetes. *Diabetes Care* 2007; **30**: 263–9.

4. Bolli GB, Gerich JE. The dawn phenomenon: a common occurrence in both non-insulin dependent and insulin dependent diabetes mellitus. *N Engl J Med* 1984; **310**: 746–50.

5. Kahn SE, Haffner SM, Heise MA *et al*: ADOPT Study Group. Glycaemic durability of rosiglitazone, metformin, or glyburide monotherapy. *N Engl J Med* 2006; **355**: 2427–43.

6. Nissen SE, Wolski K. Effect of rosiglitazone on the risk of myocardial infarction and death from cardiovascular causes. *N Engl J Med* 2007; **356**: 2457–71.

7. Krall RL. Cardiovascular safety of rosiglitazone. *Lancet* 2007; **369**: 1996–7.

8. Home PD, Pocock SJ, Beck-Nielson H *et al*. for the RECORD study group. Rosiglitazone evaluated for cardiovascular outcomes – an interim analysis. *N Engl J Med* 2007; **357**: 1–11.

9. Dormandy JA, Charbonnel B, Eckland DJ *et al*. Secondary prevention of macrovascular events in patients with type 2 diabetes in the PROactive Study (PROspective pioglitAzone Clinical Trial In macroVascular Events): a randomised controlled trial. *Lancet* 2005; **366**: 1279–89.

10. Erdmann E. The effect of pioglitazone on recurrent myocardial infarction in 2445 patients with type 2 diabetes and previous myocardial infarction – data from the PROactive study. American Heart Association, November, 2005 Dallas TX, USA.

11. Wilcox R, Bousser MG, Betteridge J *et al*. Effects of pioglitazone in patients with type 2 diabetes with or without previous stroke. Results from PROactive (PROspective pioglitAzone Clinical Trial In macroVascular Events 04). *Stroke* 2007; **38**: 865–73.

12. Ryden L, Thráinsdóttir I, Swedberg K. Adjudication of serious heart failure in patients from PROactive. *Lancet* 2007; **369**: 189–90.

List of Abbreviations

2-AG	2-arachidonoylglycerol	**CB-1**	Cannabinoid receptor-1
ACCORD	Action to Control	**CCB**	Calcium-channel blocker
	Cardiovascular Risk in Diabetes	**CHD**	Chronic heart disease
ACE	Angiotensin-converting	**CHF**	Chronic heart failure
	enzyme	**CHOIR**	Correction of Haemoglobin
ACEI	Angiotensin-converting		and Outcomes in Renal
	enzyme inhibitor		Insufficiency
ACR	Albumin:creatinine ratio	**CI**	Confidence interval
ADOPT	A Diabetes Outcome	**CKD**	Chronic kidney disease
	Progression Trial	**CLD**	Chronic liver disease
AER	Albumin excretion rate	**CrCl**	Creatinine clearance
AGE	Advanced glycosylation	**CRT**	Central retinal thickness
	end-products	**CVD**	Cardiovascular disease
ALLHAT	Antihypertensive and Lipid-		
	Lowering treatment to prevent	**DCCT**	Diabetes Control and
	Heart Attack Trial		Complications Trial
ALT	Alanine aminotransferase	**DKD**	Diabetic kidney disease
AMD	Age-related macular	**DME**	Diabetic macular oedema
	degeneration	**DPN**	Diabetic peripheral neuropathy
AMI	Acute myocardial infarction	**DPNP**	Diabetic peripheral
AMPK	AMP-activated protein kinase		neuropathic pain
ARB	Angtiotensin II receptor blocker	**DPP-4**	Dipeptidyl peptidase IV
ASCOT	Anglo–Scandinavian Cardiac	**DR**	Diabetic retinopathy
	Outcomes Trial	**DREAM**	Diabetes REduction Assessment
ASCOT-LLA	ASCOT – Lipid-Lowering Arm		with ramipril and rosiglitazone
ASCOT-BPLA	ASCOT – Blood Pressure-		Medication
	Lowering Arm		
ASPEN	Atorvastatin Study for	**eGFR:**	Estimated glomerular filtration
	Prevention of Coronary Heart		rate
	Disease Endpoints in Non-	**ELF**	European Liver Fibrosis score
	Insulin-Dependent Diabetes	**EMMACE**	Evaluation of Methods and
	Mellitus		Management of Acute
A-to-Z	Aggrastat® to Zocor®		Coronary Events
		ESA	Erythropoiesis-stimulating agent
BCVA	Best-corrected visual acuity	**ETDRS**	Early Treatment Diabetic
BMI	Body mass index		Retinopathy Study
CAD	Coronary artery disease	**FIELD**	Fenofibrate Intervention and
CARDS	Collaborative Atrovastatin		Event Lowering in Diabetes
	Diabetes Study	**FPG**	Fasting plasma glucose
CARE	Cholesterol and Recurrent		
	Events		

GI	Gastrointestinal		OCT	Optical coherence tomography
GIP	Glucose-dependent insulinotropic peptide		PCR	Protein:creatinine ratio
GLP-1	Glucagon-like peptide-1		PDR	Proliferative diabetic retinopathy
			PKC	Protein kinase C
5-HT	5-hydroxytryptamine		PKC-DRS2	PKC , Inhibitor Diabetic Retinopathy Study
Hb	Haemoglobin			
HbA1c	Glycated haemaglobin		PROactive	PROspective pioglitAzone Clinical Trial In macroVascular Events
HDL	High-density lipoprotein			
HF	Heart failure			
HOPE	Heart Outcomes Prevention Evaluation		PROVE-IT	Pravastatin or Atorvastatin Evaluation and Infection Therapy
HPS	Heart Protection Study			
HR	Hazard ratio		QA	Quality assurance
IDEAL	Incremental Decrease in End Points Through Aggressive Lipid-Lowering		RAAS	Renin–angiotensin–aldosterone system
			RCT	Randomised controlled trial
IENF	Intraepidermal nerve fibres		RECORD	Rosiglitazone Evaluated for Cardiovascular and Regulation of Glycaemia in Diabetes
IFG	Impaired fasting glucose			
IGT	Impaired glucose tolerance			
IHD	Ischaemic heart disease		ROS	Reactive oxygen species
IVTA	Intravitreal triamcinolone acetate			
			SI	Small intestine
			SMVL	Sustained moderate visual loss
JBS2	Joint British Societies 2		SNRI	Selective serotonin–noradrenalin-reuptake inhibitor
LDL	Low-density lipoprotein		SREBP	Sterol-regulatory element-binding proteins
LFT	Liver function tests			
LIPID	Long-term Intervention with Pravastatin in Ischaemic Disease		TCA	Tricyclic antodepressants
			TDI	Tissue Doppler imaging
LV	Left ventricular		TNT	Treat to New Targets
			TZD	Thiazolidinedione
MI	Myocardial infarction			
MRI	Magnetic resonance imaging		UKADS	UK Asian Diabetes Study
			UKPDS	UK Prospective Diabetes Study
NAFLD	Non-alcoholic fatty liver disease		VA	Visual acuity
NASH	Non-alcoholic steatohepatitis		VALUE	Valsartan Antihypertensive Long-term Use Evaluation
NFkB	Nuclear factor-kappa B			
NHS I, II	Nurses Health Study I,II		VEGF	Vascular endothelial growth factor
NICE	National Institute for Health and Clinical Excellence			
NNH	Number needed to harm		YAG	Yttrium aluminium garnet
NNT	Number needed to treat			
NOD	New-onset diabetes		WHO	World Health Organisation

Index